M000290844

Neurocritical Care Monitoring

Neurocritical Care Monitoring

EDITORS

Chad M. Miller, MD
Associate Professor of Neurology and Neurosurgery
Wexner Medical Center
Ohio State University
Columbus, Ohio

Michel T. Torbey, MD
Professor of Neurology and Neurosurgery
Director, Division of Cerebrovascular Diseases and Neurocritical Care
Wexner Medical Center
Ohio State University
Columbus, Ohio

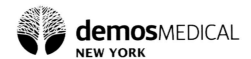

demosMEDICAL
NEW YORK

Visit our website at www.demosmedical.com

ISBN: 9781620700259
e-book ISBN: 9781617051883

Acquisitions Editor: Beth Barry
Compositor: Integra Software Services Pvt. Ltd.

© 2015 Demos Medical Publishing, LLC. All rights reserved. This book is protected by copyright. No part of it may be reproduced, stored in a retrieval system, or transmitted in any form or by any means, electronic, mechanical, photocopying, recording, or otherwise, without the prior written permission of the publisher.

Medicine is an ever-changing science. Research and clinical experience are continually expanding our knowledge, in particular our understanding of proper treatment and drug therapy. The authors, editors, and publisher have made every effort to ensure that all information in this book is in accordance with the state of knowledge at the time of production of the book. Nevertheless, the authors, editors, and publisher are not responsible for errors or omissions or for any consequences from application of the information in this book and make no warranty, expressed or implied, with respect to the contents of the publication. Every reader should examine carefully the package inserts accompanying each drug and should carefully check whether the dosage schedules mentioned therein or the contraindications stated by the manufacturer differ from the statements made in this book. Such examination is particularly important with drugs that are either rarely used or have been newly released on the market.

Library of Congress Cataloging-in-Publication Data

Neurocritical care monitoring / editors, Chad M. Miller, Michel T. Torbey.
 p. ; cm.
Includes bibliographical references and index.
ISBN 978-1-62070-025-9 (alk. paper) -- ISBN 978-1-61705-188-3 (e-book)
I. Miller, Chad M., editor. II. Torbey, Michel T., editor.
[DNLM: 1. Central Nervous System Diseases--diagnosis. 2. Neurophysiological Monitoring. 3. Critical Care--methods. 4. Nervous System Physiological Phenomena. WL 141]
RC350.N49
616.8′0428--dc23

2014032210

Special discounts on bulk quantities of Demos Medical Publishing books are available to corporations, professional associations, pharmaceutical companies, health care organizations, and other qualifying groups. For details, please contact:

Special Sales Department
Demos Medical Publishing, LLC
11 West 42nd Street, 15th Floor
New York, NY 10036
Phone: 800-532-8663 or 212-683-0072
Fax: 212-941-7842
E-mail: specialsales@demosmedical.com

Printed in the United States of America by Bradford and Bigelow.
14 15 16 17 / 5 4 3 2 1

Contents

Contributors

Latisha K. Ali, MD   Assistant Professor, Department of Neurology, UCLA
David Geffen School of Medicine, Los Angeles, California

Nessim Amin, MBBS   Fellow of Neurosciences Critical Care, Departments of
Neurological Surgery and Neurology, Wexner Medical Center, Ohio State University,
Columbus, Ohio

Enrique Carrero Cardenal, PhD   Professor, Department of Anesthesiology,
Hospital Clinic, University of Barcelona, Barcelona, Spain

Jan Claassen, MD, PhD   Assistant Professor of Neurology and Neurosurgery, Director,
Neurocritical Care Training Program, New York Presbyterian Hospital, Division of
Critical Care Neurology, Columbia University College of Physicians and Surgeons,
New York, New York

Marek Czosnyka, PhD   Professor, Department of Clinical Neurosciences, University
of Cambridge, Cambridge, United Kingdom

Andrew Demchuk, MD, FRCPC   Associate Professor, Department of Clinical
Neurosciences, University of Calgary, Calgary, Alberta, Canada

Matthew Eccher, MD, MSPH   Assistant Professor of Neurology and Neurosurgery,
Case Western Reserve University School of Medicine, Cleveland, Ohio

Romergryko Geocadin, MD   Associate Professor, Department of Anesthesiology
and Critical Care Medicine, Department of Neurology, Department of Neurosurgery,
Department of Medicine, Johns Hopkins University School of Medicine,
Baltimore, Maryland

Diana Greene-Chandos, MD   Director of Education, Quality and Outreach for Neurosciences Critical Care, Wexner Medical Center, Ohio State University, Columbus, Ohio

David S. Liebeskind, MD   Assistant Professor, Department of Neurology, UCLA David Geffen School of Medicine, Los Angeles, California

Herbert Alejandro A. Manosalva, MD   Fellow in Cerebrovascular Diseases, Movement Disorders and Neurogenetics, Department of Neurology, University of Alberta, Edmonton, Canada

Chad M. Miller, MD   Associate Professor of Neurology and Neurosurgery, Wexner Medical Center, Ohio State University, Columbus, Ohio

David M. Panczykowski, MD   Resident, Neurological Surgery, Department of Neurological Surgery, University of Pittsburgh Medical Center, Pittsburgh, Pennsylvania

Jeremy T. Ragland, MD   Fellow, Division of Neurocritical Care, Department of Neurology, Columbia University College of Physicians and Surgeons, New York Presbyterian Hospital/Columbia University Medical Center, New York, New York

Maher Saqqur, MD, MPH, FRCPC   Associate Professor, Department of Medicine, Division of Neurology, University of Alberta, Edmonton, Alberta, Canada

J. Michael Schmidt, PhD, MSc   Assistant Professor of Clinical Neuropsychology in Neurology, Informatics Director, Neurological Intensive Care Unit, Critical Care Neuromonitoring, Columbia University College of Physicians and Surgeons, New York, New York

Lori Shutter, MD   Co-Director, Neurovascular ICU, UPMC Presbyterian Hospital, Director, Neurocritical Care Fellowship, Departments of Neurology, Neurosurgery, and Critical Care Medicine, University of Pittsburgh Medical Center, Pittsburgh, Pennsylvania

Tess Slazinski, RN, MN, CCRN, CNRN, CCNS   Cedars Sinai Medical Center, Los Angeles, California

Michel T. Torbey, MD   Professor of Neurology and Neurosurgery, Director, Division of Cerebrovascular Diseases and Neurocritical Care, Wexner Medical Center, Ohio State University, Columbus, Ohio

Wei Xiong, MD   Assistant Professor of Neurology, Neurointensivist, Case Western Reserve University School of Medicine, Cleveland, Ohio

David Zygun, MD, MSc, FRCPC   Professor and Divisional Director, Departments of Critical Care Medicine, Clinical Neurosciences, and Community Health Sciences, University of Calgary, Calgary, Alberta, Canada

Foreword

When I was considering going into neurocritical care over 20 years ago, it was in large part because of an interest in the physiology (as opposed to anatomy) of acute brain catastrophes (my term), and optimism that intervention must be possible. Patients in the pulmonary and cardiac intensive care units were active, and my colleagues routinely made treatment changes many times a day based on the physiology of the patient's condition, a physiology that was identified by a monitor such as a flow-volume loop on the ventilator in an acute respiratory distress syndrome (ARDS) patient or a pulmonary-artery catheter in a patient with cardiogenic shock. As a neurology resident in an era when neurocritical care as a distinct discipline existed in very few places (my center was not one), it was interesting to watch general intensivists and neurologists alike walk past comatose patients, document an unchanged neurologic examination, declare them stable, and move on. Something nagged at me that these patients were also suffering from "active" conditions that deserved intervention. Many had suffered traumatic brain injury, ischemic stroke, intracerebral hemorrhage, and the like; if we would only identify the target, we could offer them the same level of care.

Sure, we had intracranial pressure monitoring and transcranial Doppler. I remember hearing about media reports of Dr. Randy Chesnut, who was pushing the concept that monitoring "the brain pressure" was important. We also had data from the Traumatic Coma Data Bank and Stroke Data Bank that suggested secondary brain insults were real and impacted our patients' outcomes. The *Brain Trauma Foundation Severe Head Injury Guidelines* had not yet been published, the NINDS IV t-PA study was ongoing, and the idea of directly measuring cerebral metabolism in real time made sense, but I (and my colleagues) had no idea how we might do it. Emboldened by the huge advances in basic and translational science in the 1980s and early 1990s that allowed understanding of the cellular mechanisms of acute ischemia and brain trauma, I realized that my patients were, in fact, undergoing active and potentially interveneable processes. The issue was now how to track these events and what to do.

Whenever I think I have a good new idea, I first look to the past. The relevance of cerebral metabolic function, blood flow, autoregulation, and other aspects of cerebral physiology to acute brain injury was not a new concept. Kety, Schmidt, Lassen, Fog, and others had been addressing this for nearly 60 years. It seemed that implementation science would be even more of a hurdle than the discovery of basic mechanisms had been for the emerging world of neurocritical care I was entering. If I was going to act, I needed monitors to help direct me.

I wax philosophically because I think that my experience has been similar to many other colleagues. The last 20 years have sent us on a quest to understand more deeply the active processes that may be targets for intervention in our patients. In the neurocritical care unit, physiology matters. In fact, I believe that the principal focus of neurocritical care for acute central nervous system injuries is the prevention, identification, and treatment of secondary brain and spinal cord injury. Neuromonitoring is central to this and the last two decades have seen an explosion of technical advances that allows us to assess many of the processes that we knew were going on all along. This book is timely as it provides a current perspective on many of these tools, and the molecular and physiological underpinnings that they address.

The focus of this book, on the multimodal nature of monitoring, also emphasizes one of the most important lessons we have (re)learned: we are not monitoring an individual parameter (such as cerebral blood flow, $P_{bt}O_2$, or ICP). We are monitoring a patient. Our patients are complex, with many interacting factors that all come together to define and direct their outcome from an acute neurologic catastrophe. I commend the editors for their careful perspective on the current state of neuromonitoring. The individual chapters provide excellent overviews of specific neuromonitoring tools and paradigms. Attention is paid, throughout the book, from the introduction to the final chapters, to elucidating how multimodality neuromonitoring is used by clinicians in a thoughtful way. Importantly, limitations of current technology are appropriately described and the essential role of nursing in neuromonitoring is emphasized. Also, the emerging importance of informatics technology in bringing clarity to the complexity of multimodal neuromonitoring is described.

We are at a very different place now than when I thought about going into neurocritical care. Advances in multimodal neuromonitoring have played an extremely important role in the development of the field. But as this book well describes, we are not at the end. The optimal tools and methods for improving patient outcomes remain elusive. We have made significant progress, but there is still a long way to go. I am very interested to see what I will write in the foreword to a book on *Neurocritical Care Monitoring* 20 years from now. Please enjoy this excellent book and help us all advance the field of neurocritical care.

J. Claude Hemphill III, MD, MAS, FNCS
Kenneth Rainin Endowed Chair in Neurocritical Care
Professor of Neurology and Neurological Surgery
University of California, San Francisco
President, Neurocritical Care Society

Preface

The specialty of neurocritical care arose from the identified need to provide brain-specific care to a subset of critically ill brain- and spine-injured patients. It was recognized that those patients with central nervous system injuries had unique requirements and that standard provision of critical care protocols occasionally and inadvertently disregarded those needs. Furthermore, an appreciation arose that a patient's ultimate clinical outcome often had as much to do with avoidance of clinical deterioration as it did upon the severity of the original insult. The first neurocritical care units were constructed on the premise that precise and expert physical examination could identify deterioration and allow intervention to alter the clinical course. As a result, these early units consisted of experienced and knowledgeable nurses and practitioners who focused on serial and methodical examination.

Over the past few decades, the breadth and complexity of secondary brain injury that results in patient deterioration have been better understood. Clear correlations began to be drawn between biochemical and cellular distress and eventual neuronal loss and disability. Furthermore, many of these changes were noted at stages where the patient's condition remained amenable to therapy. Coincidentally, neurointensivists began to report that care, guided by recommended general treatment parameters (eg, blood pressure, systemic arterial oxygenation etc.) was not sufficient to identify and prevent a substantial portion of secondary worsening. While treatment that considered the demands of the brain had been a therapeutic improvement, it has become clear that care directed by the specific needs of the individual patient's brain is required to optimize outcomes.

These goals have led to the heightened interest in neuromonitoring. Neuromonitoring is no longer simply a part of neurocritical care; it is essential for individualization of treatment and embodies the original intentions of the subspecialty. Utility of neuromonitoring is presently at a critical juncture, where the modifiable nature of injury is being defined and protocols utilizing the guidance of neuromonitoring devices are being tested. A detailed understanding of the various neuromonitoring devices and approaches is vital to those participating in the care of brain- and spine-injured patients.

Neurocritical Care Monitoring has been written to comprehensively address the role of neuromonitoring in neurocritical care. Current utilization, benefits, and concerns for each commercially available neuromonitoring device are discussed within the book. Additionally, basic strategies for neuromonitoring implementation and analysis are included. The editors are indebted to the contributing authors, not only for their participation in the project, but also for their contributions in advancing the field of neuromonitoring.

Intracranial Pressure Monitoring

Nessim Amin, MBBS
Diana Greene-Chandos, MD

INTRODUCTION

The roles of intracranial pressure (ICP) monitoring and control are both unique and vital to neurocritical care. When ICP rises above safe thresholds, serious consequences can ensue. As ICP rises, it decreases cerebral perfusion pressure (CPP) and may decrease cerebral blood flow (CBF) if not compensated by the intrinsic autoregulatory capacity of the brain. Additionally, persistent ICP elevations or pressure gradients bear the risk of tissue herniation and subsequent neurologic decline. Maintaining an appropriate ICP is a therapeutic principle for critical neurologically injured patients. While radiologic imaging and clinical examination of the patient can provide valuable insight regarding ICP status, ICP monitoring is required for definitive measurement and continuous tracking of this monitoring parameter.

The decision to place an invasive ICP monitor requires careful consideration, as it carries its own set of inherent risks. Furthermore, there has been recent debate regarding the appropriate indications for ICP monitoring as well as the role of ICP monitoring in improved clinical outcomes (1). Numerous noninvasive modalities have also been studied, including CT/MRI scans, fundoscopy, tympanic membrane displacement and transcranial Doppler (2), yet none have proven superior or as reliable as invasive monitoring. Despite its invasive nature, ICP monitoring via ventriculostomy has remained the gold standard for accurate measurement of ICP. Noninvasive modalities still have a place in the neurocritical care setting, as they provide further information regarding the patient's overall neurologic well-being. This chapter focuses on the invasive monitors of ICP. For critically ill brain-injured patients, ICP monitoring allows care to be tailored and individualized to meet the unique needs of the neurological or neurosurgical critical care patient.

INTRACRANIAL PRESSURE

Physiology of Intracranial Pressure Monitoring

The Monroe-Kellie doctrine states that the sum of the volume of blood, cerebrospinal fluid (CSF) and brain parenchyma must remain constant within the fixed dimensions of the rigid skull (3). These three components are essentially noncompressible and displace each other within the cranial vault to maintain a similar volume and pressure. While there is some variation in ICP and intracerebral volume associated with changes in the cardiac cycle, the ICP remains constant over the long term through compensatory decreases in the volume of one compartment when the volume of another compartment increases (4,5). This compensatory mechanism fails and intracranial hypertension ensues when an elevation in the volume of one compartment cannot be matched with an equal decrease in volume of the other two compartments.

Normal ICP tends to range between 5 and 15 mmHg, although simple coughing or sneezing can transiently elevate ICP to a pressure of 50 mmHg (6). Measuring ICP through use of a pressure transducer produces a standard waveform composed of three relatively constant peaks. The first of these three waves, the percussion wave, is derived from arterial pulsations of the large intracranial vessels (7). The second, the tidal wave, is derived from brain elasticity, and the final wave, the dicrotic wave, correlates with the arterial dicrotic notch (Figure 1.1; 8). Changes in these waves can often be the first signs of developing intracranial hypertension as cerebral compliance decreases and the arterial components become more prominent.

The failure of the compensatory mechanisms described by the Monroe-Kellie doctrine results in intracranial hypertension, which, if untreated, can lead to permanent neurologic sequelae. As ICP continues to rise, two primary problems ensue. First, elevated ICP and decreased brain elasticity increase the force exerted against arterial pressure. This, in turn, decreases cerebral perfusion pressure. While autoregulatory properties of the cerebral

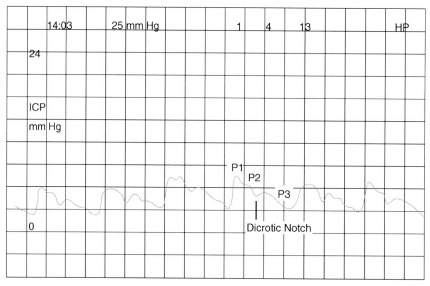

FIGURE 1.1 Graph of the component peaks of the intracranial pressure waveform.
P1 = percussion wave. P2 = tidal wave. P3 = dicrotic wave.

vasculature can compensate for this to an extent, perfusing pressures below the autoregulatory curve can ultimately lead to cerebral ischemia (9). As the volume and pressure of the contents within the fixed cranial vault increase, displacement of brain tissue results. The most profound manifestation of this displacement is brain herniation.

Initiation of an Intracranial Pressure Monitoring Device

Intracranial hypertension is found in 40% to 60% of severe head injuries and is a major factor in 50% of all fatalities. Patients with suspected elevated ICP and a deteriorating level of consciousness are candidates for invasive ICP monitoring. The Glasgow Coma Scale (GCS) level that requires ICP monitoring should be based on rate of decline and other clinical factors such as CT evidence of mass effect and hydrocephalus. In general, ICP monitors should be placed in patients with a GCS score of less than 9 and in all patients whose condition is thought to be deteriorating due to elevated ICP (level of evidence V, grade C recommendation). The type of monitor utilized depends on availability, experience, and the situation. Intraventricular ICP monitors and intraparenchymal fiberoptic ICP devices are the most commonly used methods of monitoring ICP.

ICP should be monitored in all salvageable patients with severe traumatic brain injury (TBI) with GCS 3 to 8 after resuscitation and:

(a) Abnormal CT scan of the head that reveals a hematoma, contusions, swelling, herniation, or compressed basal cisterns

(b) A normal CT scan if two or more of the following features are noted at admission: age over 40 years, unilateral or bilateral motor posturing, and systolic blood pressure less than 90 mmHg (1)

In TBI patients with a GCS greater than 8, ICP monitoring should be considered if the CT demonstrates a significant mass lesion or if treatment or sedation is required for associated injuries (13). Although ICP monitoring is widely recognized as a standard of care for patients with severe TBI, care focused on maintaining monitored ICP at 20 mmHg or less was not shown to be superior to care based on imaging and clinical examination in a recent South American study by Chesnut et al. in 2012 (1). However, in that study, there were substantial ICP lowering therapies provided to the control group and overall patient management was much different than that provided at typical North American centers.

In non traumatic settings (eg, spontaneous intracranial hemorrhage [ICH], subarachnoid hemorrhage [SAH], status epilepticus, and cerebral infarction), the decision should be individualized and based on whether elevated ICP is expected. Examples include:

(a) Spontaneous ICH:

1. Patients with a GCS score of ≤ 8, those with clinical evidence of transtentorial herniation, or those with significant intraventricular hemorrhage (IVH) or hydrocephalus might be considered for ICP monitoring and treatment. A cerebral perfusion pressure of 50 to 70 mmHg may be reasonable to maintain depending on the status of cerebral autoregulation.

2. Ventricular drainage as treatment for hydrocephalus is reasonable in patients with decreased level of consciousness (20).

(b) Aneurysmal SAH:

There are no definitive guidelines for methods and techniques for ICP management following aneurysmal SAH. Persistent ICP elevations have been correlated with poor outcomes after aneurysm rupture. Continuous ICP monitoring aids in the early detection of secondary complications and guides therapeutic intervention. (24)

ICP Thresholds

Current data support 20 to 25 mmHg as an upper threshold above which treatment is required for intracranial hypertension (21–23). There has been no difference in outcome between ICP thresholds of 20 and 25 mmHg (21). An opening ICP of 15 and higher has been identified as one of 5 factors associated with higher mortality. Brain shift and herniation result from pressure differential rather than simply height of ICP elevation. As a result, the clinical exam and imaging result should be correlated with the ICP values obtained (13).

Cerebral Perfusion Threshold

CPP is calculated as mean arterial pressure (MAP) minus ICP. Optimal CPP is typically considered to range between 50 mmHg and 70 mmHg. The TBI guidelines support a CPP > 60 (level of evidence III). Low CPP (< 55 mmHg) and systemic hypotension have been well established as predictors for death and poor outcome (12). However, aggressive attempts to elevate CPP above 70 mmHg have shown no benefit and have been associated with increased risk of acute respiratory distress syndrome (ARDS) related to the use of vasopressors and intravenous fluids (10,11). In addition, maintaining adequate CPP in patients with TBI tends to be more important than lowering ICP (11). However, it is preferred to maintain both values within the goal ranges.

Intracranial Pressure Waveforms (Lundeberg Pathological Waves)

ICP is not a static value. It exhibits cyclic variation based on the superimposed effects of cardiac contraction, respiration, and intracranial compliance. Under normal physiologic conditions, the amplitude of the waveform is often small, with B waves related to respiration and smaller C waves (or Traube-Hering-Mayer waves) related to the cardiac cycle (Figure 1.1; 25).

Pathological A waves (also called plateau waves or Lundeberg waves) are abrupt and marked elevations in ICP of 50 to 100 mmHg, which usually last minutes to hours. The presence of A waves signifies a loss of intracranial compliance, and heralds imminent decompensation of the autoregulatory mechanism. Thus, the presence of A waves should suggest the need for urgent intervention to help control ICP (Figure 1.2).

The ICP waveform is evaluated by the characteristics of each individual wave and the momentary mean ICP, as well as measures of compliance under current standard of care. However, there has been steady interest in evaluating continuous runs of ICP data for longer

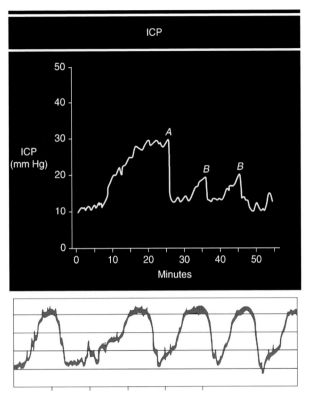

FIGURE 1.2 Pathological ICP waves. The graph in black shows an example of the Pathological A-wave (Lundberg waves) which heralds reduced intracranial compliance. The graph in white shows an example of a markedly elevated ICP near 40 mmHg with loss of the dicrotic notch.

term trends and correlations using systems and waveform analysis techniques. Goals of this type of analysis include provision of a more sensitive assessment of the pathological state and an early indicator of impending system change. These techniques have included spectral analysis, waveform correlation coefficients, and system entropy.

These analytical techniques rely on the relationship between the ICP waveform and the arterial blood pressure (ABP) waveform. The correlation coefficient between changes in ABP and ICP is defined by Cosnyka et al. (1996) as the pressure reactivity index (PRx) (9). PRx varies from low values (no association) to values approaching 1.0 (strong positive association). With lower ABP, lower blood vessel wall tension results in an increase in transmission of the ABP waveform to the ICP. Also with elevated ICP, brain compliance is reduced, thereby increasing transmission of the ABP waveform. PRx has been implicated as a marker of autoregulatory reserve.

Approximate entropy (ApEn) is a measure of system regularity/randomness, devised for use in physiological systems (63). It measures the logarithmic likelihood that runs of patterns are similar over a given number of observations. Reductions in ApEn imply reduced randomness or increased order and have been associated with pathology in the cardiovascular, respiratory, and endocrine systems. Approximate entropy analysis has been successfully applied under conditions of raised ICP for measuring changes in transmission of system randomness between the heart rate and the ICP waveform.

Duration of Monitoring

A single ICP monitoring device is used as long as clinically necessary, with reinsertion of a new monitor only if a malfunction occurs, or if CSF cultures demonstrate an infection. Routine reinsertion of a new monitor increases risk of infection by unnecessarily reexposing the patient to contamination at the time of insertion (19). There is an increased risk of infection with an external ventricular device after being in place for more than 5 days (26). Other ICP monitors (parenchymal and subdural) may begin to have measurement differences (drift) due to inability to recalibrate over time (27,28).

External ventricular drain (EVD) is both a temporary monitor and treatment option for patients with increased ICP. An EVD is usually in place for 5 to 10 days. Indications of removal include: monitoring is no longer required, infection risk is increased, hydrocephalus is resolved, and/or ventriculoperitoneal or ventriculoatrial shunt is planned. Weaning of an EVD is done with the following steps as recommended by Varelas in 2006 (29):

■ Raise the drain height by 5 cm H_2O every 12 hours only if ICP is not above the prescribed parameter.

■ When the pressure level reaches 20 cm H_2O and the EVD drains less than 200 mL/24 hours, clamp the EVD (written order obtained by neurosurgery or neurointensivist team). It is recommended to orient the stopcock "off" to drainage and "open" to the transducer. This technique is used to determine if the patient is continuing to tolerate weaning. The pressure level and the patient's clinical status postclamping guide the neurosurgical or neurointensivist team's decision to remove or unclamp the EVD.

Gradual, multistep weaning from external ventricular drainage in patients with aneurysmal SAH (aSAH) provides no advantage over rapid weaning in preventing the need for shunts. Furthermore, gradual weaning prolongs intensive care unit and hospital stays. Consequently, for aSAH patients whose EVD was placed for reasons other than ICP elevation, rapid EVD weaning may be considered rather than gradual weaning.

TYPES OF INTRACRANIAL PRESSURE MONITORING DEVICES

There are four main locations within the brain where ICP monitoring devices are frequently placed: fluid filled ventricle, brain parenchyma, subarachnoid, and epidural space. The decision of which location and device to use is based on the clinical scenario, appearance of the head CT (ie, size of cerebral lateral ventricles) and operator experience.

External Ventricular Drain EVD

Clinical Utility

1. Cerebral edema with suspected elevated ICP: This utilization is best studied in patients with TBI. However, the clinical scenario and need for an EVD can be found with SAH, non traumatic ICH, IVH, ischemic stroke, hypoxic brain injury, cerebral venous thrombosis (CVT), hepatic encephalopathy, cerebral neoplasm, and cerebral infections. EVDs not only allow monitoring of the ICP but also can serve as a treatment modality to allow drainage of CSF, which aids in lowering the ICP.

2. Hydrocephalus: Hydrocephalus occurs when there is an abnormality of production or resabsorption of CSF within and around the brain and spinal cord. The two types of hydrocephalus are communicating and obstructive. Communicating hydrocephalus occurs when CSF flow throughout the cisterns and the subarachnoid space is unimpeded. Obstructive hydrocephalus occurs when CSF flow within the ventricular system in blocked from either external compression or internal processes. In both forms of hydrocephalus, the result is an accumulation of CSF, which cannot be absorbed in a normal fashion. In acute cases where the mental status is declining, an EVD is placed and remains until the cause of the hydrocephalus is resolved. If the need for CSF diversion is persistent, ventriculo-peritoneal shunting or ventriculo-atrial shunting may be needed.

3. Surgery: Some surgical procedures of the brain are aided by draining some CSF from the ventricles. In these cases, an external ventricular drain may be placed at the start or during the procedure to drain fluid for brain relaxation (eg, in aSAH, resection of Chiari malformations, or brain tumor).

4. Administering medication: There are some conditions that may require the direct administration of medication into the cerebral ventricular system to bypass the blood–brain barrier. In order to do this, some patients may require a ventricular catheter, which enables intrathecal injection. Common clinical scenarios where the ventriculostomy has been used to inject medications include antibiotic administration for bacterial ventriculitis (31), intrathecal chemotherapy for brain cancer (32), and tissue plasminogen activator injection for clearance of IVH (33). These catheters can be used while the patient is in the hospital. However, when patients require long-term treatment, a permanent catheter can be placed, which is connected to a reservoir under the scalp called an Omaya reservoir. This is most commonly used for chemotherapeutic agents or antibiotics for refractory ventriculitis.

Anatomy and Placement

The gold standard technique for ICP monitoring is a catheter inserted into the lateral ventricle, usually via a small right frontal burr hole. Under aseptic conditions, a scalp incision is made over the insertion site. Commonly, the Kocher's point is used, which is located 2.5-cm lateral to the midline (or at the midpupillary line), 11-cm posterior to the nasion. To avoid the motor cortex, it should be at least 1-cm anterior to the coronal suture. A burr hole is then performed. After opening the dura, a ventricular catheter is passed into the ipsilateral lateral ventricle transcerebrally. This may be done free-handedly or under the guidance of ultrasound or neuronavigation software. After confirming CSF drainage, the distal end of the catheter is tunneled subcutaneously and allowed to exit the skin approximately 5 cm from the burr hole site. The catheter is connected to a closed external drainage system with an attached ICP monitoring transducer. Though clear benefit has not been demonstrated, prophylactic antibiotics can be given perioperatively to reduce the risk of infection.

(a) Fluid-Coupled monitor EVD (detailed figure shown in Figure 1.4)

This monitoring system connects to the bedside patient monitor with a pressure cable plugged into a designated pressure module. The benefit of fluid-coupled systems is the ability to zero the device after insertion. However, these devices may require the nurse to recalibrate at intervals after the system is in use and is highly dependent upon accurate leveling to the tragus. The transducer is rezeroed after a shift (minimally every 12 hours), as a troubleshooting technique, or when interface with the monitor has been interrupted. The transducer should not require rezeroing when repositioning the patient (Figures 1.3, 1.4, and 1.5) but rather appropriate releveling.

(b) Air-Coupled monitor EVD (Hummingbird -Figure 1.6)

This device senses pressure by utilizing a proprietary bladder filled with air. This unique technology carries pressure waves in the air-coupled system on the terminal end of the patient monitoring cable. The leveling problems inherent in the fluid-filled monitors are eliminated resulting in precise and artifact-free, high-fidelity waveform that does not require releveling with patient movement. The bladder is connected to an air–fluid lumen that terminates into the air-pulse luer. When the air-coupled system is cycled, air is removed and a small amount of air is replaced charging the air-coupled ICP system. The transducer/cable does not require leveling and can be zeroed in situ (Figure 1.6).

Advantages/Disadvantages
The overall advantages of either type of EVD are that it measures global ICP while allowing for drainage of CSF for both diagnostic and therapeutic purposes. It has the ability to be calibrated externally in the fluid-coupled device. The air-coupled device allows for continuous CSF drainage and continuous monitoring, which cannot be done with the fluid-coupled device. The fluid-coupled EVD requires that the drainage be stopped to transmit an accurate pressure wave. The fluid-coupled device is dependent on accurate leveling of

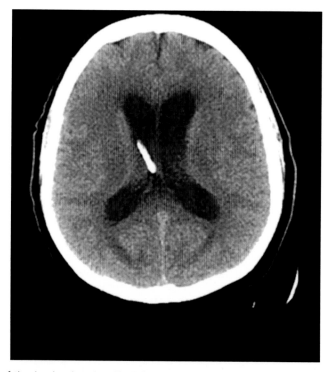

FIGURE 1.3 CT of the brain showing EVD fluid-coupled monitor.

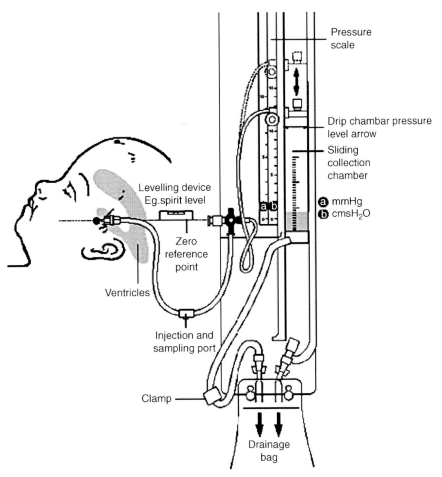

FIGURE 1.4 Example of a fluid-coupled EVD. The transducer is leveled to the tragus of the patient.

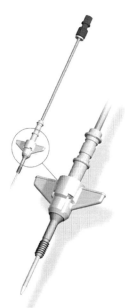

FIGURE 1.5 Example of air-coupled EVD catheter.

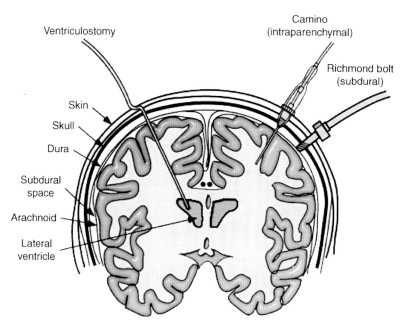

FIGURE 1.6 Diagram showing examples of an intraparenchymal monitor, Richmond bolt, and ventriculostomy in place.

the device for an accurate pressure, whereas the air-coupled device does not. Both devices allow for administration of drugs (eg, antibiotics, chemotherapeutic agents).

The disadvantages of an EVD is that it is the most invasive of all of the ICP monitoring options. Depending on the skill of the operator, multiple passes through the brain parenchyma may be required to enter the ventricular system. Each pass through the parenchyma increases the risk of an EVD track hematoma resulting in further brain damage (30). An EVD is also difficult to place if there is ventricular effacement or displacement due to brain swelling or intracranial mass lesions. If the ventricles are too effaced, then use of an alternate ICP device should be considered (ie, intraparenchymal monitor). Care also should be taken with EVDs when mass effect is present. EVDs have the potential to worsen side-to-side shift by drainage of the ventricle opposite mass effect and can cause an upward herniation syndrome from rapid drainage in the setting of elevated posterior fossa pressure due to a mass, hemorrhage, or edema. In one study, the use of an EVD was associated with an infection rate of 11%. The most common infection pathogens are *Staphylococcus epidermidis* and *Staphylococcus aureus*. As many as 25% of infections are caused by gram-negative organisms such as *Escherichia coli*, *Acinetobacter*, and *Klebsiella* species (34). Occlusion of the catheter with blood and debris is another complication that can be corrected with gentle flushing using low volume (1 mL) preservative-free saline. Each injection into the ventricular system increases the risk of infection (35).

Intraparenchymal Intracranial Pressure Monitor

Intraparenchymal monitoring devices consist of a thin cable with an electronic or fiberoptic transducer at the tip. These monitors can be inserted directly into the brain parenchyma via a small hole drilled in the frontal skull under sterile conditions.

Anatomy and Placement

The monitor is placed in the right or left prefrontal area. The most injured side should be selected in a focal injury. In diffuse brain injury or edema, the right hemisphere is generally used.

Advantages/Disadvantages

The advantages of an intraparenchymal ICP monitor include the ease of placement, low morbidity, and the ability to add additional monitoring probes such as brain tissue oxygen monitor (LICOX), cerebral blood flow (HEMEDEX), and cerebral microdiaysis probes to a multilumen bolt. It also carries lower risk of infection than EVDs and a lower nursing task burden.

The disadvantages include the inability to drain CSF for diagnostic or therapeutic purposes and the potential to lose accuracy (or "drift") over several days, since the transducer cannot be recalibrated following initial placement. In addition, there is a greater risk of mechanical failure due to the complex design of these monitors (15–18).

Subarachnoid Intracranial Pressure Monitor

This is another fluid-coupled system that connects the intracranial space to an external transducer at the bedside via saline-filled tubing. The subarachnoid bolt is actually a hollow screw that is inserted via a burr hole. The dura at the base of the bolt is perforated with a spinal needle, allowing the subarachnoid CSF to fill the bolt. Pressure tubing is then connected to establish communication with a pressure monitoring system. This method of ICP monitoring is no longer commonly used. The advantages include its minimally invasive nature and a low risk of infection.

The disadvantages include decreased accuracy compared to the intraventricular or intraparenchymal monitors; blockage of the system by tissue debris and increased cerebral edema; need for frequent recalibration; and increased risk of bleeding into the subarachnoid space.

Epidural Intracranial Pressure Monitors

This device (the Gaeltec device) is inserted into the inner table of the skull and superficial to the dura. Typically, pressure is transduced by an optical sensor. These have a low infection rate (approximately 1%) but are prone to malfunction, displacement, and baseline drift that can exceed 5 ± 10 mmHg after more than a few days of use. Much of the inaccuracy results from having the relatively inelastic dura between the sensor tip and the subarachnoid space.

Epidural monitors contain optical transducers that rest against the dura after passing through the skull. They often are inaccurate, as the dura dampens the pressure transmitted to the epidural space and, thus, are of limited clinical utility. They have been most commonly used in the setting of coagulopathic patients with hepatic encephalopathy whose course is complicated by cerebral edema. In this setting, use of these catheters is associated with a significantly lower risk of ICH (4% vs 20% and 22%, respectively, for intraparenchymal and intraventricular devices). It is also associated with decreased fatal hemorrhages (1% vs 5% and 4%, respectively, for intraparenchymal and intraventricular devices; 14). Otherwise, this device is rarely used in clinical practice.

Lumbar Catheter Intracranial Pressure Monitoring

Lumbar drainage devices (LDDs) are closed sterile systems that allow the drainage of CSF from the subarachnoid space. LDDs are inserted via a specialized spinal needle, known as a Touhy needle, into the lumbar subarachnoid space at the L2–L3 level or below. This placement avoids injury to the spinal cord, which ends at the conus medullaris at the level of the L1–L2 vertebral bodies. In the lumbar CSF space, the flexible spinal catheter will lie alongside the cauda equina, which consists of the ventral and dorsal spinal nerve roots that descend from the spinal cord and exit the spinal canal at lumbosacral levels. Insertion of the spinal catheter may cause transient radicular pain if the catheter brushes against one of the spinal nerve roots.

Occasionally, the pain can be persistent, especially if lumbar spinal stenosis causes the spinal catheter and the spinal nerve roots to remain in close contact. Placement of an LDD is an accepted medical therapy for the treatment of postoperative or traumatic dural fistulae (ie, CSF leak), treatment of shunt infections, and for the diagnostic evaluation of idiopathic normal pressure hydrocephalus. LDDs also are used to reduce ICP during a craniotomy and as adjuvant therapy in the management of traumatically brain-injured patients.

Additional Concerns With Intracranial Pressure Monitoring Devices

Antibiotic Prophylaxis

The patients at greater risk for ICP monitor–related infection include those with the following features: prolonged monitoring greater than 5 days, presence of ventriculostomy vs intraparenchymal monitor, CSF leak, concurrent infection, or serial ICP monitor placements. Multiple studies support the use of prophylactic systemic antibiotics throughout the duration of external ventricular drainage. However, prophylactic use of antibiotics raises concern for an increase in bacterial antimicrobial resistance. Recent studies have shown that antibiotics treatment given only during the insertion of the EVD may be associated with comparable infectious risks. The use of antibiotic-coated EVDs to prevent ventriculitis has proven to be effective (36) in one study; however, the use of a silver-impregnated catheter was not proven to be beneficial (36,37).

Deep Venous Thrombosis Prophylaxis

Chemical prophylaxis has been shown to decrease rates of venous thrombosis formation and subsequent pulmonary embolism in neurologically critically ill patients. The incidence of bleeding was not different between early (24 hours) and delayed (72 hours) administration of chemical prophylaxis in relation to insertion of either an EVD or intraparenchymal device, but there was reduced incidence of deep vein thrombosis (DVT)/pulmonary embolism (PE) with early administration. In addition, the early start of chemical prophylaxis did not show an increase in hemorrhagic complications (60).

Dressing and Dressing Changes of the EVD

Skilled nursing is key to minimizing complications related to external ventricular drains. Dressing of the EVD site must be observed hourly to ensure that a CSF leak has not occurred. If a leak is identified, the insertion site should be inspected and the dressing should be replaced. Dressings should be changed using sterile technique when visibly soiled (61). Incorrect or asterile dressing change has been associated with increased risk for ventriculitis (62).

Antiplatelet and Anticoagulant Use With EVDs

There is a trend toward higher bleeding complications from EVD placement in patients who are on antiplatelet or anticoagulant therapy. When starting these agents, one must weigh the indication for the agent with the risk of a ventriculostomy track hematoma or intraparenchymal monitor–associated bleed. The early use of chemical, subcutaneously injected, VTE chemoprophylaxis (first 24 hours) did not increase the incidence of bleeding complications but did not show better protection against venous thromboembolism when compared to delayed administration (64).

CRITICAL CARE MANAGEMENT OF ELEVATED INTRACRANIAL PRESSURE

General Measures

The head and neck should be optimally positioned to minimize additional elevations in ICP. The head of the bed should be elevated to 30 degrees for patients with poor intracranial compliance. The neck should be free from compression, and the head should be positioned in the midline. When a cervical collar is present, it should be fitted just tight enough to provide stability but not so tight as to cause internal jugular vein compression.

Normorthermia (36–38°C) is strongly recommended in patients with cerebral edema, irrespective of the underlying etiology, to avoid the deleterious effects of fever on outcome (38). Numerous clinical trials have reported the value of induced moderate hypothermia for ICP control (39). Hyperthermia will increase ICP (40). Control of fever includes administration of acetaminophen (325–650 mg orally or rectally every 6 hours) or ibuprofen (400 mg orally every 6 hours). In addition, surface cooling with ice packs, cool blankets, or surface devices (Artic Sun) is an effective noninvasive way to reduce fever. Intravascular cooling devices utilize a catheter with a balloon that circulates fluid internally; it is inserted into the inferior vena cava via the femoral vein, thereby allowing access to the body's internal circulation to change temperature when that flow interacts with the catheter. It has been shown to be a highly effective, quick, and precise form of temperature control, but it does carry a procedural risk, increased risk of venous thrombosis (41), and risk of infection from a central venous catheter. (42)

Maintenance of euvolemia (with 0.9 % normal saline) is essential. Mild hypervolemia can be considered in order to maintain CPP, but this needs to be done judiciously to avoid pulmonary edema and ARDS. Hypotonic fluids such as 0.45% saline and dextrose in water should be avoided (43).

Normocarbia (PaCO$_2$ 35–45 mmHg) is preferred because hypercarbia will add to elevations in ICP resulting from cerebral vasodilitation. In addition, avoidance of hypoxemia and maintenance of PaO$_2$ of 100 mg are recommended.

Agitation contributes to elevated ICP. Care must be taken to ensure that pain is addressed adequately with short-acting narcotics such as morphine and fentanyl. Alcohol, illicit drug withdrawal, and delirium should be considered if pain is not responsible. When required, short-acting sedative agents are always preferred for the neurological population so that an adequate examination can still be obtained.

The use of prophylactic anti epileptic drugs (AEDs) remains controversial in the setting of acute brain injury. Seizures, whether they are clinically evident or nonconvulsive, result in elevations of ICP (44). AED prophylaxis in patients with TBI may be given for 1 week, but there is no evidence to support routine continued use (45). In patients with ICH or SAH, AEDs should not be routinely initiated, unless it is thought that a seizure might result in rehemorrhage or worsening of an unprotected aneurysm. Corticosteroids are beneficial only for patients with vasogenic edema related to abscess or brain tumors.

Specific Measures

Hyperventilation is very effective in reducing ICPs related to cerebral edema acutely and for a short period of time (46). It works via the vasoconstrictor effect of decreased $PaCO_2$, which persists only for 10 to 20 hours. $PaCO_2$ levels below 25 can increase the risk of secondary cerebral ischemia from too much vasoconstriction (47). Sustained hyperventilation for 5 days has been shown to slow recovery of severe TBI at 3 and 6 months (48,49).

The use of osmotic therapy or hypertonic saline (HTS) is an effective way to reduce ICP from cerebral edema. For osmotic therapy, mannitol can be used with a target serum osmolality of 300 to 320 (50). It is administered as a 0.25 to 1.5 g/kg bolus intravenously. Mechanisms of action include acute dehydrating effect and secondary hyperosmolality (diuretic effect). Side effects include hypotension, hypovolemia, and renal tubular damage. Hypertonic saline boluses and infusions (3%, 7.5 %, 10%, and 23.4 %) have proven to be effective in numerous clinical scenarios marked by ICH. HTS administered in bolus form can resolve ICP episodes refractory to mannitol (51). The most effective concentrations and protocols for HTS use require further study.

The use of barbiturates results from their ability to reduce brain metabolism and cerebral blood flow, thus lowering ICP. Barbiturate use may also exert a neuroprotective effect (52). Pentobarbital is most commonly used, with a loading dose of 5 to 20 mg/kg as a bolus, followed by 1 to 4 mg/kg per hr infusion. Barbiturate therapy can be complicated by hypotension, possibly requiring vasopressor support. The use of barbiturates is also associated with a loss of the neurologic examination, and requires accurate ICP, hemodynamic, and often EEG monitoring to guide therapy

As discussed earlier, a ventriculostomy should be inserted for very specific criteria for specific disease states. Rapid drainage of CSF should be avoided because this may lead to subdural hemorrhage (53). A lumbar drain is generally contraindicated in the setting of high ICP due to the risk of transtentorial herniation or central herniation.

When all medical measures to control ICH fail, decompressive hemi-craniectomy (DHC) can be considered. DHC removes the rigid confines of the bony skull, allowing noncompressive expansion of the volume of the intracranial contents. There is a growing body of literature supporting the efficacy of decompressive craniectomy in certain clinical situations. Importantly, it has been demonstrated that in patients with elevated ICP, craniectomy alone lowered ICP 15%, but opening the dura in addition to the bony skull resulted in an average decrease in ICP of 70% (54,55). Decompressive craniectomy also appears to improve brain tissue oxygenation (56). It has been shown to improve outcomes in malignant MCA stroke syndromes (57), but has not been shown to improve outcomes in TBI (58,59).

REFERENCES

1. Chesnut RM et al. A trial of intracranial-pressure monitoring in traumatic brain injury. *N Engl J Med.* 2012;367(26):2471–2481.
2. Raboel PH et al. Intracranial Pressure Monitoring: Invasive versus Non-Invasive Methods-A Review. *Crit Care Res Pract.* 2012;2012: 1–14.
3. Monro A. *Observations on the Structure and Functions of the Nervous System* 1783, Edinburgh: Printed for, and sold by, W. Creech. 176 p.
4. Greitz D et al. Pulsatile brain movement and associated hydrodynamics studied by magnetic resonance phase imaging. The Monro-Kellie doctrine revisited. *Neuroradiology.* 1992;34(5):370–380.
5. Neff S and Subramaniam RP, Monro-Kellie doctrine. *J Neurosurg.* 1996;85(6):1195.
6. Winn HR and Youmans JR. *Youmans Neurological Surgery.* 2004;5th:[4 v. (lxiv, 5296, cviii) ill. (some col.) 28 cm. + 1 CD-ROM (4 3/4 in.)].
7. Cardoso ER, Rowan JO, Galbraith S. Analysis of the cerebrospinal fluid pulse wave in intracranial pressure. *J Neurosurg.* 1983;59(5):817–821.
8. Hamer J et al. Influence of systemic and cerebral vascular factors on the cerebrospinal fluid pulse waves. *J Neurosurg.* 1977;46(1):36–45.
9. Marion DW, Darby J, Yonas H. Acute regional cerebral blood flow changes caused by severe head injuries. *J Neurosurg.* 1991;74(3):407–414.
10. Schmidt JM et al. Cerebral perfusion pressure thresholds for brain tissue hypoxia and metabolic crisis after poor-grade subarachnoid hemorrhage. *Stroke.* 2011;42(5):1351–1356.
11. Rosner MJ, Rosner SD, Johnson AH. Cerebral perfusion pressure: management protocol and clinical results. *J Neurosurg.* 1995;83(6):949–962.
12. Balestreri M et al. Impact of intracranial pressure and cerebral perfusion pressure on severe disability and mortality after head injury. *Neurocrit Care.* 2006;4(1):8–13.
13. Brain Trauma Foundation; American Association of Neurological Surgeons; Congress of Neurological Surgeons; Joint Section on Neurotrauma and Critical Care, AANS/CNS, Bratton SL, Chestnut RM, Ghajar J, McConnell Hammond FF, Harris OA, Hartl R, Manley GT, Nemecek A, Newell DW, Rosenthal G, Schouten J, Shutter L, Timmons SD, Ullman JS, Videtta W, Wilberger JE, Wright DW. Guidelines for the management of severe traumatic brain injury. VI. Indications for intracranial pressure monitoring. *J Neurotrauma.* 2007;24 Suppl 1:S37–S44.
14. Blei AT, Olafsson S, Webster S, et al. Complications of intracranial pressure monitoring in fulminant hepatic failure. *Lancet.* 1993;341:157.
15. Ostrup RC, Luerssen TG, Marshall LF, et al. Continuous monitoring of intracranial pressure with a miniaturized fiberoptic device. *J Neurosurg.* 1987;67:206.
16. Gambardella G, d'Avella D, Tomasello F. Monitoring of brain tissue pressure with a fiberoptic device. *Neurosurgery.* 1992;31:918.
17. Bochicchio M, Latronico N, Zappa S, et al. Bedside burr hole for intracranial pressure monitoring performed by intensive care physicians. A 5-year experience. *Intensive Care Med* 1996;22:1070.
18. Kasotakis G, Michailidou M, Bramos A, et al. Intraparenchymal vs extracranial ventricular drain intracranial pressure monitors in traumatic brain injury: less is more? *J Am Coll Surg.* 2012 Jun;214(6):950–957. doi: 10.1016/j.jamcollsurg.2012.03.004. Epub 2012 Apr 26.
19. Kantar RK, Weiner LB, Patti AM, et al. Infectious complications and duration of intracranial pressure monitoring. *Crit Care Med.* 1985 Oct;13(10):837–839.
20. Morgenstern LB, Hemphill JC III, Anderson C, et al. American Heart Association Stroke Council and Council on Cardiovascular Nursing. Guidelines for the management of spontaneous intracerebral hemorrhage: a guideline for healthcare professionals from the American Heart Association/American Stroke Association. *Stroke.* 2010 Sep;41(9):2108–2129. doi: 10.1161/STR.0b013e3181ec611b. Epub 2010 Jul 22.

21. Ratanalert S, Phuenpathom N, Saeheng S, et al. ICP threshold in CPP management of severe head injury patients. *Surg Neurol.* 2004 May;61(5):429–434; discussion 434–435.

22. Saul TG, Ducker TB. Effect of intracranial pressure monitoring and aggressive treatment on mortality in severe head injury. *J Neurosurg.* 1982 Apr;56(4):498–503.

23. Narayan RK et al. Intracranial pressure: to monitor or not to monitor? A review of our experience with severe head injury. *J Neurosurg.* 1982 May;56(5):650–659.

24. Mack WJ, King RG, Ducruet AF, et al. Intracranial Pressure Following Aneurysmal Subarachnoid Hemorrhage: Monitoring Practices and Outcome Data. *Neurosurg Focus.* 2003;14(4).

25. Hayashi M, Handa Y, Kobayashi H, et al. Plateau-wave phenomenon (I). Correlation between the appearance of plateau waves and CSF circulation in patients with intracranial hypertension. *Brain.* 1991;114 (Pt 6):2681.

26. Rebuck, K. Murry, D. Rhoney, D. et al. Infection related to intracranial pressure monitors in adults: analysis of risk factors and antibiotic prophylaxis. *J Neurol Neurosurg Psychiatry.* 2000 September;69(3):381–384.

27. Chen L, Du HG, Yin LC, et al. Zero drift of intraventricular and subdural intracranial pressure monitoring systems. *Chin J Traumatol.* 2013;16(2):99–102.

28. Rosa M Martínez-Mañasa, David Santamartab, José M de Camposb, et al. Camino® intracranial pressure monitor: prospective study of accuracy and complications. *J Neurol Neurosurg Psychiatry* 2000;69:82–86.

29. Varelas P, Helms A, Sinson G, et al. Clipping or coiling of ruptured cerebral aneurysms and shunt-dependent hydrocephalus. *Neurocrit Care.* 2006;4(3):223–228.

30. Maniker AH, Vaynman AY, Karimi RJ, et al. Hemorrhagic complications of external ventricular drainage. *Neurosurgery.* 2006 Oct;59(4 Suppl 2):ONS419-24; discussion ONS424-5.

31. Mueller SW, Kiser TH, Anderson TA, et al. Intraventricular daptomycin and intravenous linezolid for the treatment of external ventricular-drain-associatedventriculitis due to vancomycin-resistant Enterococcus faecium. *Ann Pharmacother.* 2012 Dec;46(12):e35. doi: 10.1345/aph.1R412. Epub 2012 Dec 11.

32. Birnbaum T, Baumgarten LV, Dudel C, et al. Successful long-term control of lymphomatous meningitis with intraventricular rituximab. *J Clin Neurosci.* 2013 Sep 17. pii: S0967-5868(13) 00287-7.

33. Ziai W, Moullaali T, Nekoovaght-Tak S, Ullman N, et al. No exacerbation of perihematomal edema with intraventricular tissue plasminogen activator in patients with spontaneous intraventricular hemorrhage. *Neurocrit Care.* 2013 Jun;18(3):354–361.

34. Beer R, Lackner P, Pfausler B, et al. Nosocomial ventriculitis and meningitis in neurocritical care patients. *J Neurol.* 2008 Nov;255(11):1617–1624.

35. Hill M, Baker G, Carter D, et al. A multidisciplinary approach to end external ventricular drain infections in the neurocritical care unit. *J Neurosci Nurs.* 2012 Aug;44(4):188–193.

36. Sonabend AM, Korenfeld Y, Crisman C, et al. Prevention of ventriculostomy-related infections with prophylactic antibiotics and antibiotic-coated external ventricular drains: a systematic review. *Neurosurgery.* 2011 Apr;68(4):996–1005.

37. Xiang Wang, Yan Dong, Xiang-Qian Qi, et al. Clinical review: Efficacy of antimicrobial-impregnated catheters in external ventricular drainage—a systematic review and meta-analysis. *Critical Care* 2013, 17:234.

38. Rossi S, Zanier ER, Mauri I, et al. Brain temperature, body core temperature, and intracranial pressure in acute cerebral damage. *J Neurol Neurosurg Psychiatry.* 2001 Oct;71(4):448–454.

39. Polderman KH. Induced hypothermia and fever control for prevention and treatment of neurological injuries. Lancet 2008;371:1955–1969.

40. Jiang JY, Xu W, Li WP, et al. Effect of long-term mild hypothermia or short-term mild hypothermia on outcome of patients with severe traumatic brain injury. *J Cereb Blood Flow Metab.* 2006;26:771–776.

41. Simosa HF, Petersen DJ, Agarwal SK, et al. Increased risk of deep venous thrombosis with endovascular cooling in patients with traumatic head injury. *Am Surg.* 2007 May;73(5):461–464.

42. Patel N, Nair SU, Gowd P, et al. Central line associated blood stream infection related to cooling catheter in cardiac arrest survivors undergoing therapeutic hypothermia by endovascular cooling. *Conn Med.* 2013 Jan;77(1):35–41.

43. Zornow MH, Prough DS. Fluid management in patients with traumatic brain injury. *New Horiz.* 1995 Aug;3(3):488–498.

44. Gabor AJ, Brooks AG, Scobey RP, et al. Intracranial pressure during epileptic seizures. *Electroencephalogr Clin Neurophysiol.* 1984 Jun;57(6):497–506.

45. Chang BS, Lowenstein DH; Quality Standards Subcommittee of the American Academy of Neurology. Practice parameter: antiepileptic drug prophylaxis in severe traumatic brain injury: report of the Quality Standards Subcommittee of the American Academy of Neurology. *Neurology.* 2003 Jan 14;60(1):10–16.

46. Heffner JE, Sahn SA. Controlled hyperventilation in patients with intracranial hypertension. Application and management. *Arch Intern Med.* 1983 Apr;143(4):765–769.

47. Yundt KD, Diringer MN. The use of hyperventilation and its impact on cerebral ischemia in the treatment of traumatic brain injury. *Crit Care Clin.* 1997 Jan;13(1):163–184.

48. Diringer MN, Videen TO, Yundt K, et al. Regional cerebrovascular and metabolic effects of hyperventilation after severe traumatic brain injury. *J Neurosurg.* 2002 Jan;96(1):103–108.

49. Muizelaar JP, Marmarou A, Ward JD, et al. Adverse effects of prolonged hyperventilation in patients with severe head injury: a randomized clinical trial. *J Neurosurg.* 1991 Nov;75(5):731–739.

50. Roberts I, Schierhout G, Wakai A. Mannitol for acute traumatic brain injury. *Cochrane Database Syst Rev.* 2003;(2):CD001049

51. Fisher B, Thomas D and Peterson B. Hypertonic saline lowers raised intracranial pressure in children after head trauma. *J Neurosurg Anesthesiol.* 1992;4:4–10.

52. Roberts I. Barbiturates for acute traumatic brain injury. *Cochrane Database Syst Rev.* 2000;(2):CD000033.

53. Andrade AF, Paiva WS, Amorim RL, et al. Continuous ventricular cerebrospinal fluid drainage with intracranial pressure monitoring for management of posttraumatic diffuse brain swelling. *Arq Neuropsiquiatr.* 2011 Feb;69(1):79–84.

54. Timofeev I, Czosnyka M, Nortje J, et al. Effect of decompressive craniectomy on intracranial pressure and cerebrospinal compensation following traumatic brain injury. *J Neurosurg.* 2008 Jan;108(1):66–73.

55. Kunze E, Meixensberger J, Janka M, et al. Decompressive craniectomy in patients with uncontrollable intracranial hypertension. *Acta Neurochir Suppl.* 1998;71:16–18.

56. M Jaeger, M Soehle, and J Meixensberger. Effects of decompressive craniectomy on brain tissue oxygen in patients with intracranial hypertension. *J Neurol Neurosurg Psychiatry.* 2003 April; 74(4):513–515

57. Yang XF, Yao Y, Hu WW, et al. Is decompressive craniectomy for malignant middle cerebral artery infarction of any worth? *J Zhejiang Univ Sci B.* 2005 Jul;6(7):644–649.

58. D. J. Cooper, J. V. Rosenfeld, L. Murray, et al. Decompressive craniectomy in diffuse traumatic brain injury. *The New England Journal of Medicine*, vol. 364, no. 16, pp. 1493–1502, 2011.

59. J. Ma, C. You, L. Ma, et al. Is decompressive craniectomy useless in severe traumatic brain injury? *Critical Care*, vol. 15, no. 5, article 193, 2011.

60. Tanweer O, Boah A, Huang PP. Risks for hemorrhagic complications after placement of external ventricular drains with early chemical prophylaxis against venous thromboembolisms . *J Neurosurg.* 2013 Nov;119(5):1309–1313.

61. Slazinski. T. et al. Care of the patient undergoing intracranial pressure monitoring/external ventricular drainage or lumbar drainage. *American Association of Neuroscience Nurses*: 1–37.

62. Korinek AM, Reina M, Boch AL, et al. Prevention of external ventricular drain-related ventriculitis. *Acta Neurochir (Wien).* 2005 Jan;147(1):39-45; discussion 45–46.

63. Pincus SM. Approximate entropy as a measure of system complexity. *Proc Natl Acad Sci U S A* 1991 March 15;88(6):2297–2301.

64. Tanweer O, Boah A, Huang PP. Risks for hemorrhagic complications after placement of external ventricular drains with early chemical prophylaxis against venous thromboembolisms. *J Neurosurg.* 2013 Nov;119(5):1309–1313.

2

Transcranial Doppler Monitoring

Maher Saqqur, MD, MPH, FRCPC
David Zygun, MD, MSc, FRCPC
Andrew Demchuk, MD, FRCPC
Herbert Alejandro A. Manosalva, MD

INTRODUCTION

Transcranial Doppler (TCD) has been increasingly utilized as a monitoring tool in the neurocritical care unit (NCCU) because it is a noninvasive tool and can be brought to the bedside.

The purpose of this chapter is to provide an account of the common indications for TCD in the NCCU. The number one indication for TCD in the NCCU is the detection and monitoring of vasospasm (VSP) in patients with aneurysmal and traumatic subarachnoid hemorrhage (SAH). In addition, TCD is being studied as a noninvasive estimator of intracranial pressure (ICP) and cerebral perfusion pressure (CPP) in patients with severe traumatic brain injury (TBI). In addition, TCD has been utilized as a monitoring tool for detection of microembolic signals in the presence of acute ischemic stroke. Finally, TCD has been extensively studied in the setting of clinical brain death.

Over the past decade, Power M-Mode TCD, transcranial color coded duplex, and the use of contrast agents have extended the utility of TCD in the NCCU to include indications such as monitoring of arterial occlusion in acute ischemic stroke and detection of microembolic signals in carotid stenosis and cardioemboli disease (1).

SUBARACHNOID HEMORRHAGE: DETECTION OF VASOSPASM

Cerebral VSP is a delayed narrowing of the cerebral vessels that is induced by blood products that remain in contact with the cerebral vessel wall following SAH (2). VSP usually begins about day 3 after onset of SAH and is maximal by day 6 to 8. It is often responsible for delayed cerebral ischemia (DCI) seen in SAH patients (3). In addition, patients with severe VSP have a significantly higher mortality than those without VSP. The most common cause of SAH is the spontaneous rupture of a cerebral aneurysm (4). Other causes include head injury and neurosurgical procedures such as brain tumor resection. VSP resulting from aneurysmal SAH is a well-known complication, occurring in up to 40% of patients after an aneurysmal SAH, and carries a 15% to 20% risk of stroke or death (5).

VSP was first demonstrated angiographically by Ecker and Riemenschneider as cerebral arterial narrowing following SAH (6). Cerebral angiography of the brain is considered the gold standard for detection of VSP. However, this procedure is invasive and carries the risk of complications such as stroke due to cerebral embolus, dissection, or rupture of cerebral arteries (7). Almost 20 years ago, TCD was proposed for the diagnosis of cerebral VSP (8). The diagnosis of spasm with a TCD device is based on the hemodynamic principle that the velocity of blood flow in an artery is inversely related to the area of the lumen of that artery. In theory, TCD may serve as a relatively simple screening method of cerebral VSP, and some investigators have advocated the replacement of angiography by TCD (9–11).

While TCD is effective in identifying VSP, several studies have demonstrated that isolated use of TCD flow velocity numbers cannot accurately assess the presence of VSP, whereas repeated series of TCD measurements may enhance the diagnostic accuracy of this tool (12).

TECHNICAL ASPECTS OF TRANSCRANIAL DOPPLER

TCD is a noninvasive, bedside, transcranial US method of determining flow velocities in the basal cerebral arteries. When using a range-gated Doppler US instrument, placement of the probe in the temporal area just above the zygomatic arch allows the velocities in the middle cerebral artery (MCA) to be determined from the Doppler signals. The flow velocities in the proximal anterior (ACA), terminal intracranial artery (tICA) and posterior (PCA) cerebral arteries can be recorded at steady state and during test compression of the common carotid arteries.

TCD monitoring often begins by obtaining a baseline TCD study on day 2 or 3 post-SAH onset with adherence to a comprehensive isonation protocol, which examines all proximal intracranial arteries. TCD studies are then continued daily from day 4 to day 14 after SAH onset. The TCD examination begins with temporal window isonation of the proximal MCA on the affected side, usually 50 to 60 mm, and then distal MCA, at a depth of 40 to 50 mm. The examination then returns proximally to the MCA/ACA bifurcation, where a bidirectional flow signal is located at 60 to 80 mm depth. The temporal window isonation continues with more caudal angulation of the probe to evaluate the tICA at 60 to 70 mm depth. The temporal window isonation is completed by posterior angulation to evaluate the PCA at depth 55 to 75 mm. The protocol is then repeated for the opposite hemisphere. The ICA siphon can also be isonated via the transorbital window at depths of 60 to 70 mm. This is preferable if no temporal ICA signal can be obtained.

The transforaminal window isonation occurs via the foramen magnum and is first performed at 75 mm depth to locate the terminal vertebral artery (VA) and proximal basilar artery (BA). Isonation of the BA is performed distally along its course (range 80 to 100 mm depth), followed by assessment of the more proximal left and right VAs at depths of 50 to 80 mm by lateral probe positioning. Finally, submandibular window isonation is performed to obtain reference velocities from the cervical internal carotid artery (cICA) for calculation of the Lindegaard ratio. The Lindegaard ratio, or hemispheric index, compares the highest velocity recorded in an intracranial vessel divided by the highest velocity recorded in the ipsilateral extracranial ICA.

TCD technology called Power M-mode TCD (PMD/TCD) is now available and simplifies operator dependence of TCD by providing multigate flow information simultaneously in the PMD display (1). PMD/TCD is attractive as a rapid bedside technology since PMD facilitates temporal window location and alignment of the US beam to enable assessment of multiple vessels simultaneously, without sound or spectral clues. The presence of signal drop-off with PMD as a result of excess turbulence can indicate flow disturbance resulting from VSP (Figure 2.1; 13).

The degree of VSP in the basal vessels is correlated with the amount of acceleration of blood flow velocities through the vessels as they become narrowed (11). The greatest correlation between TCD MFV and angiographic vessel narrowing occurs in the MCA. Lindegaard et al (11) showed that the vasospastic MCA usually demonstrates velocities greater than 120 cm/sec on TCD with the velocities being inversely related to arterial diameter. In

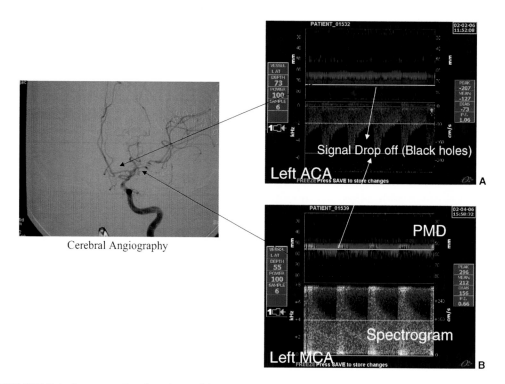

FIGURE 2.1 An example of patient with severe left MCA and moderate ACA VSP: The highest MFVs were obtained at the drop-off signals in both MCA and ACA vessels.

(A) Left ACA MFV = 127 cm/sec is an indicative of moderate VSP.
(B) Left MCA MFV = 212 cm/sec is an indicative of severe VSP.

addition, velocities greater than 200 cm/sec are predictive of a residual MCA lumen diameter of 1 mm or less. The normal MCA diameter is approximately 3 mm.

Unfortunately, TCD mean flow velocities (MFVs) do not allow calculation of cerebral blood flow (CBF) volume and cannot be substituted for CBF measurements (14–16). The TCD MFV provides a prediction assessment of the degree of vessel narrowing, spasm progression or regression, and compensatory vasodilatation.

TCD has been used as monitoring tool for the development of cerebral VSP in different drugs trials (17,18). It has also been utilized to monitor the efficacy of interventional angioplasty treatment (19) and to detect the recurrence of arterial narrowing (20).

While elevated TCD MFVs can suggest cerebral VSP, the velocities alone cannot determine if a patient has symptomatic cerebral VSP (21). In addition, different intracranial vessels have different velocity criteria for diagnosing VSP. In the next few sections, we review the literature for TCD criteria for different intracranial vessels.

A recent study by Kantelhardt et al showed that CT angiography can be easily and efficiently compared to TCD. It can provide anatomic orientation of the trajectory of the artery and may help to standardize investigation protocols and reduce inter investigator variability. In addition, image guidance may also allow extension of the use of TCD to situations of a pathological or variant vascular anatomy (22).

Middle Cerebral Artery Vasospasm

TCD has a well-documented and established value in detecting MCA VSP (MCA-VSP) (23–29). The TCD sensitivity varies from 38% to 91% and the specificity varies from 94% to 100%. (See Figure 2.1 as an example of a patient with severe proximal MCA and ACA VSP.)

Vora et al (28) studied the correlation between proximal MCA MFV and angiographic VSP after SAH. They explored three different parameters: MCA highest MFV at three depths (5, 5.5, 6 cm), the largest MFV increase in 1 day before digital subtraction cerebral angiography (DSA), and ipsilateral MCA/cotralateral MCA MFV difference. For MCA MFV ≥ 120 cm/sec, the sensitivity of TCD for detecting moderate or severe MCA VSP was 88% and the specificity was 72%. Whereas for MCA MFV ≥ 200 cm/sec, the sensitivity of TCD for detecting moderate or severe MCA-VSP was 27% and the specificity is 98%. So, for individual patients, only low or very high middle cerebral artery flow velocities (ie, < 120 or ≥ 200 cm/s) reliably predicted the absence or presence of clinically significant angiographic VSP (moderate or severe VSP). Intermediate velocities, which were observed in approximately one-half of the patients, were not dependable and should be interpreted with caution. Interestingly, all patients with MCA MFV 160 to 199 cm/sec and right-to-left MFV difference > 40 cm/sec have significant VSP.

Burch et al (23) found TCD had low sensitivity (43%) but good specificity (93.7%) for detecting moderate or severe VSP (> 50%) when MCA MFV 120 cm/sec was used as the cut-off. When the diagnostic criterion was changed to at least 130 cm/sec, specificities were 100% (tICA) and 96% (MCA) and positive predictive values were 100% (tICA) and 87% (MCA). The authors conclude that TCD accurately detects tICA and MCA-VSP when flow velocities are at least 130 cm/sec. However, its sensitivity may be underestimated and the importance of operator error overestimated.

Finally, increased blood flow velocities (FV) may not necessarily denote arterial narrowing. Both increasing flow and reduced vessel diameter may lead to high FVs. Consequently, cerebral VSP may not be differentiated from cerebral hyperemia by the mere assessment of FV in the basal arteries (27,28). To account for this diagnostic shortcoming of TCD, Lindegaard et al (10) suggested defined use of ratios of FVs between intracranial arteries and cervical internal carotid artery (ICA). The normal value for this ratio is 1.7 + 0.4. (30). It is recommended to use each patient as his or her own control since there are anatomical differences among individuals. The presence of a MCA/cervical ICA MFV ratio > 3 is indicative of moderate proximal MCA VSP, whereas a ratio > 6 is an indicative of severe VSP.

MCA VSP detection is influenced by multiple factors: improper vessel identification (tICA, PCA), increased collateral flow, hyperemia/hyperperfusion, proximal hemodynamic lesion (cervical ICA stenosis or occlusion), operator inexperience, and aberrant vessel course.

Recently, our group derived TCD criteria for detecting MCA-VSP to facilitate more accurate detection of VSP based on angiographic proven MCA-VSP. On the basis of our study's findings, (31) we proposed a TCD scoring system for the detection of MCA-VSP. Using single criterion, only moderate sensitivity and specificity for VSP detection can be achieved. In our study, we showed that combining multiple criteria (baseline MCA MFV ≥ 120, preangio MCA MFV ≥ 150, and the ratio of preangio MCA MFV to baseline MCA MFV ≥ 1.5) resulted in better accuracy for MCA-VSP detection (31) (Figure 2.2).

Anterior Cerebral Artery Vasospasm

The ability of TCD to detect anterior cerebral artery VSP (ACA-VSP) has been examined in different studies (8,24,26,32,33). In general, TCD has low sensitivity (13%–83%) and moderate specificity (65%–100%) for detecting ACA-VSP.

Wozniak et al (33) found that TCD has very low sensitivity (18%) but good specificity (65%) for detecting any degree of ACA-VSP. She used the ACA MFV > 120 cm/sec as criterion for VSP. For moderate and severe VSP (> 50% stenosis), the sensitivity increased to 35%. Grollimund and colleagues (32), using the FV criteria of a 50% increase in ACA-FVs, accurately detected VSP in 10 out of 14 subjects (sensitivity 71%). ACA-VSP could not be detected when it was present in the more distal pericallosal portions of the ACA. In contrast, Lennihan and coworkers (26) used a FV criteria of at least 140 cm/sec and detected VSP in only 2 out of 15 ACAs (sensitivity 13%). VSP was present in a portion of five ACAs not insonated by TCD. Doppler signals could not be isonated from nine ACAs (false-positive occlusion), including three ACAs with angiographic VSP. Aaslid and coauthors found that FVs in ACAs correlated poorly with residual lumen diameter.

ACA VSP detection can be limited by the presence of collateral flow (a patient with one ACA VSP might not have high MFV in that affected vessel since flow will be diverted

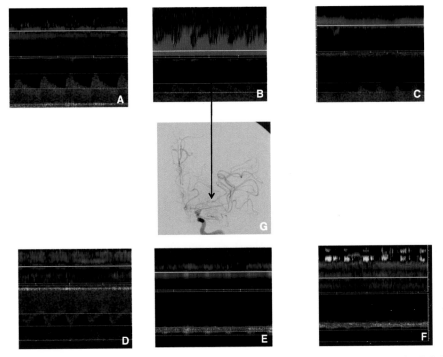

FIGURE 2.2 52-year-old patient who underwent endovascular coil embolization for left ICA saccular aneurysm.

(A) Day2: baseline TCD showing left MCA MFV 136 cm/sec (bMCA MFV ≥ 120)

(B) Day 6: preangio left MCA MFV 210 cm/sec (aMCA/ bMCA MFV ratio = 1.55) showing preangio MCA MFV > 150 and aMCA/bMCA MFV ratio ≥ 1.5

(C) Day 6: preangio right MCA MFV 99 cm/sec (aMCA/cMCA MFV ratio = 1.4) showing aMCA/cMCA MFV ratio ≥ 1.25

(D) Day 6: preangio left ACA MFV of 168 cm/sec (aMCA/(i)ACA MFV ratio = 1.5)

(E) Day 6: preangio left PCA MFV of 32 cm/sec (aMCA/iPCA MFV ratio = 8) showing aMCA/ iPCA MFV ratio ≥ 2.5

(F) Day 6: preangio left ICA (extracranial) MFV of 30 cm/sec (aMCA Lindegaard Ratio = 8.6) showing aMCA Lindegaard Ratio ≥ 3

(G) Day 6: cerebral angiography showing left MCA severe VSP

to the contralateral ACA through the Acomm), difficulty isonating the more distal A2 segment (pericallosal artery), and poor angle of isonation in the temporal window.

Internal Carotid Artery Vasospasm

There are few studies that examined the role of TCD in detecting ICA-VSP (23,34).

Burch et al (23) found that when a MFV of at least 90 cm/sec was used to indicate terminal ICA (tICA) VSP, the sensitivity was 25% and specificity was 93%. When the diagnostic criterion was changed to at least 130 cm/sec, specificities were 100% (iICA) and 96% (MCA), and positive predictive values were 100% (iICA) and 87% (MCA). The authors conclude that TCD accurately detects tICA and MCA vasospasm when flow velocities are at least 130 cm/sec. However, its sensitivity may be underestimated and the importance of operator error overestimated.

ICA VSP detection is affected by several factors: increased collateral flow, hyperemia/hyperperfusion, and anatomical factors (angle of insonation between the trajectories of ophthalmic artery (OA) and vasospasm ICA > 30 degrees).

Vertebral and Basilar Arteries Vasospasm

The ability of TCD to detect vertebral basilar artery VSP (VB-VSP) has been examined in numerous studies (35–37).

Sloan and coworkers (36) found that MFV ≥ 60 cm/sec was indicative of both vertebral (VA) and basilar artery (BA) vasospasm. For the VA, the sensitivity was 44% and specificity was 87.5%. For the BA, the sensitivity was 76.9% and specificity was 79.3%. When the diagnostic criterion was changed to ≥ 80 cm/sec (VA) and ≥ 95 cm/sec (BA), all false-positive results were eliminated (specificity and positive predictive value, 100%). He concluded that TCD has good specificity for the detection of VA VSP and good sensitivity and specificity for the detection of BA VSP. TCD is highly specific (100%) for VA and BA VSP when flow velocities are ≥ 80 and ≥ 95 cm/sec, respectively.

Soustiel et al (37) found that the BA:extracranial vertebral artery (eVA) ratio may contribute to an improved discrimination between BA VSP and vertebrobasilar hyperemia, while enhancing the accuracy and reliability of TCD in the diagnosis of BA VSP. BA:eVA threshold value of three accurately delineates patients suffering from high-grade BA VSP (50% diameter reduction).

The difficulty in detecting VB VSP can be caused by multiple factors, which include severe bilateral PCA VSP, increased collateral flow, hyperperfusion, and anatomical variations (horizontal course of VA, tortuous course of BA).

Complete TCD Examination with Lindegaard Ratio Determination

Although TCD identificaton of MCA VSP is most accurate, an isonation protocol studying all basilar vessels demonstrates greater diagnostic impact than sole MCA isonation (34). Naval et al (12) performed a two-part study designed to compare the reliability of relative increases in flow velocities with conventionally used absolute flow velocity indices and to correct for hyperemia-induced flow velocity change. Relative changes in flow velocities in patients with aneurysmal SAH correlated better with clinically significant VSP than absolute flow velocity indices. Correction for hyperemia (Lindegaard Ratio) improved predictive value of TCD in VSP. All ten patients who developed symptomatic VSP exhibited a twofold increase in flow velocities prior to developing symptomatic VSP. Five patients had a threefold increase.

Distal Vasospasm Detection by TCD

VSP can be limited to a distal vascular pattern in a small percentage of cases. Distal VSP is often not detected by TCD (38). Its occurrence can be anticipated by distal distribution of blood on posthemorrhage head CT. In some circumstances, reduced flow in the M2 segment can be picked up on TCD and is suggestive of distal narrowing. Fortunately, isolated distal VSP is a rare entity (38) and cerebral blood flow methods such as xenon CT or SPECT are useful in confirming the diagnosis. Newer CT angiography bolus techniques provide better delineation of the distal vasculature.

TCD monitoring is advantageous since it is portable, inexpensive, easily repeatable, and noninvasive. However, there is some limitation due to operator dependence and insensitivity for detecting distal vasospasm. TCD appears to have the greatest value in detecting MCA VSP, although a complete intracranial artery evaluation should be performed with use of the Lindegaard Ratio to correct for hyperemia-induced flow velocity change. In addition, trending and day-to-day comparisons of blood flow velocities are critical in identifying VSP. An MFV increase of 50 cm/sec or more during the first 24-hour period is indicative of a high risk of delayed cerebral ischemia due to VSP (39).

TRANSCRANIAL DOPPLER IN TRAUMATIC BRAIN INJURY: INTRACRANIAL PRESSURE AND CEREBRAL PERFUSION PRESSURE

The measurement and management of ICP, in conjunction with CPP, is recommended in patients following severe traumatic brain injury (40,41). Conventionally, ICP measurement has required placement of an invasive monitor. These monitors carry the risk of infection, hemorrhage, malfunction, obstruction, or malposition. Consequently, TCD has been suggested as a potential noninvasive assessment of ICP and CPP.

A number of different approaches have been employed to describe the relationship among TCD parameters, CPP, and ICP. Chan and colleagues studied 41 patients with severe TBI (42). As ICP increased and CPP decreased, flow velocity fell. This fall preferentially affected diastolic values initially. Below a CPP threshold of 70 mmHg, they found a progressive increase in the TCD pulsatility index [PI = (peak systolic velocity – end-diastolic velocity)/timed mean velocity] ($r = -0.942$, $P < .0001$). This occurred whether the CPP decrease was due to an increase in ICP or a decrease in arterial blood pressure. Klingelhofer showed that increasing ICPs are reflected in changes in the Pourcelot index (peak systolic velocity – end-diastolic velocity/peak systolic velocity) and MFV (43). In a subsequent study, the same group demonstrated a good correlation between ICP and the product mean systemic arterial pressure × Pourcelot index/MFV in a select group of 13 patients with cerebral disease ($r = 0.873$; $P \le .001$) (44). Homberg found PI changes 2.4% per mmHg ICP (45).

Although the aforementioned evidence suggests TCD parameters are correlated with ICP and CPP in certain instances, acceptance into clinical practice requires analysis of agreement of noninvasive estimation methods with measured values. Initial proposed formulas for the prediction of absolute CPP have proved disappointing with large 95% confidence intervals (CI) for predictors (46,47). Schmidt and colleagues showed that a prototype bilateral TCD machine with a built in algorithm to assess CPP and externally measured values for arterial blood pressure has improved correlation with invasively measured perfusion (48). They used the formula CPP = mean arterial blood pressure × diastolic flow velocity/MFV + 14 mmHg and found the absolute difference between measured CPP and estimated CPP was less than 10 mmHg in 89% of measurements and less than 13 mmHg in 92% of measurements. The 95% CI range for predictors was ± 12 mmHg for the CPP, varying from 70 to 95 mmHg. Attempts at estimation of ICP have demonstrated similar CIs (49). Unfortunately, these values are still unacceptable for clinical purposes. Bellner and colleagues determined pulsatility index correlation with ICP (> 20 mmHg) to have a sensitivity of 0.89 and specificity of 0.92 (50). They concluded PI may provide guidance in those patients with suspected intracranial hypertension and repeated measurements may be of use in the NCCU.

Finally, TCD has role as a monitoring tool for cerebral vasospasm after TBI. Its occurrence is variable and can be seen in 19% to 68% of the cases. However, the clinical course tends to be milder, with earlier onset and shorter duration in comparison to aneurysmal SAH (51). In recent study by Razumovsky et al in wartime TBI, he found TCD signs of mild, moderate, and severe VSPs were observed in 37%, 22%, and 12% of patients, respectively. TCD signs of intracranial hypertension were recorded in 62.2%, of which five patients (4.5%) underwent transluminal angioplasty for posttraumatic clinical vasospasm treatment and 16 (14.4%) had a craniectomy. He concluded that cerebral arterial spasm and intracranial hypertension are frequent and significant complications of combat TBI. Therefore, daily TCD monitoring is recommended for their recognition and subsequent management (52).

BRAIN DEATH

TCD findings compatible with the diagnosis of brain death include: (a) brief systolic forward flow or systolic spikes with diastolic reversed flow, (b) brief systolic forward flow or systolic spikes and no diastolic flow, or (c) no demonstrable flow in a patient in whom flow had been clearly documented on a previous TCD examination. Recently, de Freitas and Andre performed a systematic review of 16 previous studies examining the use of TCD in patients with the clinical diagnosis of brain death (64). The overall sensitivity was 88% with the most common cause of false negatives being a lack of signal in 7% and persistence of flow in 5%. The overall specificity was 98%. Importantly, the criteria for brain death was variable, with only seven groups assessing the vertebrobasilar artery and some authors accepting the absence of flow in only one artery. The same authors performed the largest study to date including 206 patients with the clinical diagnosis of brain death in Brazil. TCD had a sensitivity of 75% for confirming brain death. Multivariable analysis revealed absence of sympathomimetric drug use and female gender were associated with false negative results. The validity of TCD diagnosed brain death depends on the time lapse between brain death and the performance of TCD (65), as some patients require repeated examinations before TCD criteria are met (66).

Acute Ischemic Stroke and Monitoring of Recanalization

Ultra-early neuroimaging may provide crucial information for the individual patient by determining the status of arterial occlusion and collateral perfusion, as well as the extent and severity of ischemia in the earliest stages of treatment (67). Noncontrast computed tomography (NCCT) can provide information regarding the extent and severity of ischemic injury by visualization of early ischemic changes. Hyperdense MCA stem and the M2 MCA "dot" sign (68) give some clues to the location of the occlusion and clot burden. CT angiography (CTA) and MR angiography (MRA) are available modalities to assess vessel patency in acute stroke (69–70). However, both imaging methods are "snapshots in time" and are unable to provide continuous information about arterial patency during or after intravenous tPA treatment. TCD is ideal for such bedside monitoring. It is inexpensive, portable, noninvasive, and requires minimal patient cooperation. TCD has not been widely accepted for use in acute stroke because of the belief that TCD is too operator dependent to be applied to acute stroke decision making. Several studies have compared TCD with digital subtraction (DSA), CTA, and MRA in the acute stroke setting with variable accuracy (71–74). Utilization of detailed diagnostic TCD criteria using specific flow findings demonstrates that accuracy can be improved. TCD accuracy for detection of MCA occlusion is superior to other intracranial locations such as VA and BA occlusions (75,76).

The PMD/TCD appears to improve window detection and simplifies operator dependence of TCD by providing multi gate flow information simultaneously in the Power M-mode display (1). PMD/TCD facilitates temporal window location and alignment of the US beam to view blood flow from multiple vessels simultaneously, without sound or spectral clues (Figure 2.3; 78).

Prolonged TCD monitoring has been performed for years. No adverse biological effects have ever been documented for the frequencies and power ranges used in diagnostic US if applied according to safety guidelines (79). Recent work has demonstrated a role for TCD monitoring in acute stroke to follow the evolution of the MCA occlusion in real time (80) and to determine the speed of clot lysis (81). Obtaining continuous information about the status of an arterial occlusion in acute stroke has the potential to be very helpful in further decision making with thrombolytic therapy (82). Some sites of arterial occlusion

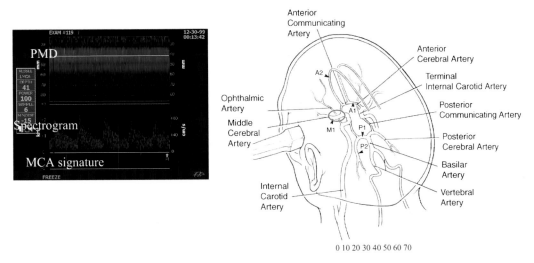

FIGURE 2.3 Trans-temporal window: MCA M1 and M2 signatures are obtained by aiming the probe anterior between the ear and frontal process of zygomatic bone, using 100% US power at 30 to 60 mm depth.

have been demonstrated to have a limited response to tPA. Terminal ICA and tandem ICA/ MCA arterial occlusions are less likely to recanalize completely (83).

The timing of arterial recanalization after IV rt-PA therapy, as determined with TCD, correlates with clinical recovery from stroke and demonstrates a 300-minute window to achieve early complete recovery (84). Rapid arterial recanalization is associated with better short-term improvement, whereas slow (> 30 minutes) flow improvement and dampened flow signal are associated with a less favorable prognosis (85). Overall, degree of recanalization by TCD is an independent predictor of outcome. When combined with stroke severity and early CT ischemic change, it is most predictive of early outcome after intravenous tPA administration (86). Early reocclusion is another common finding of TCD monitoring during thrombolysis, which complicates systemic tPA therapy. Up to 34% of tPA-treated patients with recanalization develop reocclusion. This accounted for two thirds of patients who deteriorated clinically after initial improvement (87,88).

Monitoring for Emboli

TCD is able to detect high-intensity transient signals (HITS), otherwise referred to as microembolic signals (MES), which represent emboli traversing through the major intracranial vessels (Figure 2.4). MES correspond to true emboli in animal models (89). TCD can monitor for emboli by continuous isonation of the middle cerebral arteries bilaterally. These MES are frequently early following an acute stroke (90). Microembolic signals represent an

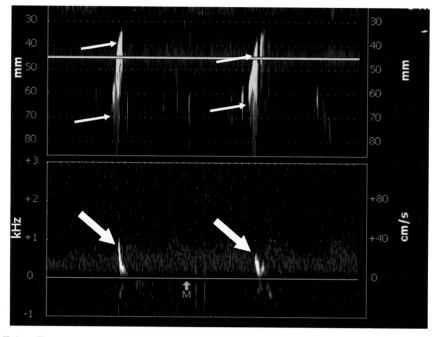

FIGURE 2.4 Two microembolic signals displaying high intensity, brief duration, and unidirection on spectrogram (white thick arrows) and movement over time across space on mmode (white thin arrows).

independent predictor of early ischemic recurrence when the cause appears related to large artery atherosclerosis such as carotid or middle cerebral artery stenosis (91–95). Emboli detection has also be shown to optimize the management of carotid endarterectomy with reduced emboli counts after postoperative dextran therapy (96). Similarly, emboli monitoring during carotid stenting demonstrated lower emboli counts with a proximal endovascular clamping when compared to a filter device (97).

Acetylsalicylic acid (98–99), clopidogrel, (100) and tirofiban/heparin (101) all appear effective in reducing MES counts and have shown trends to reductions in clinical ischemic events (TIA/stroke). Combinations of these therapies seem most effective at abolishing microembolization. Large-scale trials are needed with clinical outcomes as the primary endpoint.

Carotid Endarterectomy and Carotid Artery Stenting

TCD monitoring during carotid endarterectomy can provide information regarding the flow velocities in the MCA segment that correlate with the stump pressure during surgical cross clamping. In addition, TCD can provide real-time monitoring of MES during carotid endarterectomy (CEA) and carotid stenting, and these results have been correlated with the occurrence of new ischemic stroke.

SUMMARY

TCD is an established monitoring modality in the NCCU. It is a validated screening test for the diagnosis of vasospasm in patients with subarachnoid hemorrhage and may be used to follow therapy. Recent evidence suggests TCD holds promise for the detection of critical elevations of ICP and decreases in CPP. TCD findings of brain death are well described and its use may allow for the most favorable timing of the confirmatory test such as angiography. Finally, TCD has a defined role in acute ischemic stroke as both a diagnostic and monitoring tool.

REFERENCES

1. Moehring MA, Spencer MP. Power m-mode Doppler (pmd) for observing cerebral blood flow and tracking emboli. *Ultrasound in medicine & biology.* 2002;28:49–57.
2. Weir B, Grace M, Hansen J, Rothberg C. Time course of vasospasm in man. *J Neurosurg.* 1978;48:173–178.
3. Sloan M. Cerebral vasoconstriction: Physiology, patho-physiology and occurrence in selected cerebrovascular disorder. In: Caplan LR, ed. *Brain ischemia : Basic concept and their clinical relevance.* London: Springer-Verlag; 1994:151–172.
4. Reynolds AF, Shaw CM. Bleeding patterns from ruptured intracranial aneurysms: An autopsy series of 205 patients. *Surg Neurol.* 1981;15:232–235.
5. Bleck TP. Rebleeding and vasospasm after sah: New strategies for improving outcome. *J Crit Illn.* 1997;12:572–582.
6. Ecker A, Riemenschneider PA. Arteriographic demonstration of spasm of the intracranial arteries, with special reference to saccular arterial aneurysms. *J Neurosurg.* 1951;8:660–667.
7. Cloft HJ, Joseph GJ, Dion JE. Risk of cerebral angiography in patients with subarachnoid hemorrhage, cerebral aneurysm, and arteriovenous malformation: A meta-analysis. *Stroke.* 1999;30:317–320.
8. Aaslid R, Huber P, Nornes H. Evaluation of cerebrovascular spasm with transcranial Doppler ultrasound. *J Neurosurg.* 1984;60:37–41.

9. Seiler R, Grolimund P, Huber P. Transcranial Doppler sonography. An alternative to angiography in the evaluation of vasospasm after subarachnoid hemorrhage. *Acta radiologica. Supplementum.* 1986;369:99–102.

10. Lindegaard KF, Nornes H, Bakke SJ, et al. Cerebral vasospasm diagnosis by means of angiography and blood velocity measurements. *Acta Neurochir (Wien).* 1989;100:12–24.

11. Lindegaard KF, Nornes H, Bakke SJ, et al. Cerebral vasospasm after subarachnoid haemorrhage investigated by means of transcranial Doppler ultrasound. *Acta Neurochir Suppl (Wien).* 1988;42:81–84.

12. Naval NS, Thomas CE, Urrutia VC. Relative changes in flow velocities in vasospasm after subarachnoid hemorrhage: A transcranial Doppler study. *Neurocritical care.* 2005;2:133–140.

13. Akhtar N, Saqqur M, Roy J, et al. Developing criteria on power m mode transcranial Doppler ultrasound for angiographic proven cerebral vasospasm in aneurysmal subarachnoid hemorrhage patients. *World Stroke Congress (abstract).* 2004.

14. Yonas H, Sekhar L, Johnson DW, et al. Determination of irreversible ischemia by xenon-enhanced computed tomographic monitoring of cerebral blood flow in patients with symptomatic vasospasm. *Neurosurgery.* 1989;24:368–372.

15. Clyde BL, Resnick DK, Yonas H, et al. The relationship of blood velocity as measured by transcranial Doppler ultrasonography to cerebral blood flow as determined by stable xenon computed tomographic studies after aneurysmal subarachnoid hemorrhage. *Neurosurgery.* 1996;38:896–904; discussion 904–905.

16. Romner B, Brandt L, Berntman L, et al. Simultaneous transcranial Doppler sonography and cerebral blood flow measurements of cerebrovascular CO_2-reactivity in patients with aneurysmal subarachnoid haemorrhage. *British journal of neurosurgery.* 1991;5:31–37.

17. Yahia AM, Kirmani JF, Qureshi AI, et al. The safety and feasibility of continuous intravenous magnesium sulfate for prevention of cerebral vasospasm in aneurysmal subarachnoid hemorrhage. *Neurocritical care.* 2005;3:16–23.

18. Pachl J, Haninec P, Tencer T, et al. The effect of subarachnoid sodium nitroprusside on the prevention of vasospasm in subarachnoid haemorrhage. *Acta neurochirurgica. Supplement.* 2005;95:141–145.

19. Newell DW, Eskridge JM, Mayberg MR, et al. Angioplasty for the treatment of symptomatic vasospasm following subarachnoid hemorrhage. *J Neurosurg.* 1989;71:654–660.

20. Hurst RW, Schnee C, Raps EC, et al. Role of transcranial Doppler in neuroradiological treatment of intracranial vasospasm. *Stroke.* 1993;24:299–303.

21. Torbey MT, Hauser TK, Bhardwaj A, et al. Effect of age on cerebral blood flow velocity and incidence of vasospasm after aneurysmal subarachnoid hemorrhage. *Stroke.* 2001;32:2005–2011.

22. Kantelhardt SR, Greke C, Keric N, et al. Image guidance for transcranial Doppler ultrasonography. *Neurosurgery.* 2011;68:257–266; discussion 266.

23. Burch CM, Wozniak MA, Sloan MA, et al. Detection of intracranial internal carotid artery and middle cerebral artery vasospasm following subarachnoid hemorrhage. *Journal of neuroimaging: official journal of the American Society of Neuroimaging.* 1996;6:8–15.

24. Kyoi K, Hashimoto H, Tokunaga H, et al. [time course of blood velocity changes and clinical symptoms related to cerebral vasospasm and prognosis after aneurysmal surgery]. *No Shinkei Geka.* 1989;17:21–30.

25. Langlois O, Rabehenoina C, Proust F, et al. [diagnosis of vasospasm: Comparison between arteriography and transcranial Doppler. A series of 112 comparative tests]. *Neurochirurgie.* 1992;38: 138–140.

26. Lennihan L, Petty GW, Fink ME, et al. Transcranial Doppler detection of anterior cerebral artery vasospasm. *J Neurol Neurosurg Psychiatry.* 1993;56:906–909.

27. Sloan MA, Haley EC, Jr., Kassell NF, et al. Sensitivity and specificity of transcranial Doppler ultrasonography in the diagnosis of vasospasm following subarachnoid hemorrhage. *Neurology.* 1989;39:1514–1518.

28. Vora YY, Suarez-Almazor M, Steinke DE, et al. Role of transcranial Doppler monitoring in the diagnosis of cerebral vasospasm after subarachnoid hemorrhage. *Neurosurgery.* 1999;44:1237–1247; discussion 1247–1248.

29. Hutchison K, Weir B. Transcranial Doppler studies in aneurysm patients. *The Canadian journal of neurological sciences. Le journal canadien des sciences neurologiques*. 1989;16:411–416.

30. Aaslid R, Markwalder TM, Nornes H. Noninvasive transcranial Doppler ultrasound recording of flow velocity in basal cerebral arteries. *J Neurosurg*. 1982;57:769–774.

31. Sebastian J, Derksen C, Khan K, et al. Derivation of transcranial Doppler criteria for angiographically proven middle cerebral artery vasospasm after aneurysmal subarachnoid hemorrhage. *Journal of neuroimaging : official journal of the American Society of Neuroimaging*. 2013;23:489–494.

32. Grolimund P, Seiler RW, Aaslid R, et al. Evaluation of cerebrovascular disease by combined extracranial and transcranial Doppler sonography. Experience in 1,039 patients. *Stroke*. 1987;18:1018–1024.

33. Wozniak MA, Sloan MA, Rothman MI, et al. Detection of vasospasm by transcranial Doppler sonography. The challenges of the anterior and posterior cerebral arteries. *Journal of neuroimaging: official journal of the American Society of Neuroimaging*. 1996;6:87–93.

34. Creissard P, Proust F. Vasospasm diagnosis: Theoretical sensitivity of transcranial Doppler evaluated using 135 angiograms demonstrating vasospasm. Practical consequences. *Acta neurochirurgica*. 1994;131:12–18.

35. Soustiel JF, Bruk B, Shik B, et al. Transcranial Doppler in vertebrobasilar vasospasm after subarachnoid hemorrhage. *Neurosurgery*. 1998;43:282–291; discussion 291–293.

36. Sloan MA, Burch CM, Wozniak MA, et al. Transcranial Doppler detection of vertebrobasilar vasospasm following subarachnoid hemorrhage. *Stroke*. 1994;25:2187–2197.

37. Soustiel JF, Shik V, Shreiber R, et al. Basilar vasospasm diagnosis: Investigation of a modified "lindegaard index" based on imaging studies and blood velocity measurements of the basilar artery. *Stroke: a journal of cerebral circulation*. 2002;33:72–77.

38. Newell DW, Grady MS, Eskridge JM, et al. Distribution of angiographic vasospasm after subarachnoid hemorrhage: Implications for diagnosis by transcranial Doppler ultrasonography. *Neurosurgery*. 1990;27:574–577.

39. Grosset DG, Straiton J, du Trevou M, et al. Prediction of symptomatic vasospasm after subarachnoid hemorrhage by rapidly increasing transcranial Doppler velocity and cerebral blood flow changes. *Stroke: a journal of cerebral circulation*. 1992;23:674–679.

40. The Brain Trauma Foundation. The American Association of Neurological Surgeons. The joint section on neurotrauma and critical care. Indications for intracranial pressure monitoring. *J Neurotrauma*. 2000;17:479–491.

41. The Brain Trauma Foundation. The American Association of Neurological Surgeons. The joint section on neurotrauma and critical care. Guidelines for cerebral perfusion pressure. *J Neurotrauma*. 2000;17:507–511.

42. Chan KH, Miller JD, Dearden NM, et al. The effect of changes in cerebral perfusion pressure upon middle cerebral artery blood flow velocity and jugular bulb venous oxygen saturation after severe brain injury. *J Neurosurg*. 1992;77:55–61.

43. Klingelhofer J, Conrad B, Benecke R, et al. Intracranial flow patterns at increasing intracranial pressure. *Klin Wochenschr*. 1987;65:542–545.

44. Klingelhofer J, Conrad B, Benecke R, et al. Evaluation of intracranial pressure from transcranial Doppler studies in cerebral disease. *J Neurol*. 1988;235:159–162.

45. Homburg AM, Jakobsen M, Enevoldsen E. Transcranial Doppler recordings in raised intracranial pressure. *Acta Neurol Scand*. 1993;87:488–493.

46. Czosnyka M, Matta BF, Smielewski P, et al. Cerebral perfusion pressure in head-injured patients: A noninvasive assessment using transcranial Doppler ultrasonography. *J Neurosurg*. 1998;88:802–808.

47. Aaslid R, Lundar T, Lindegaard KF. Estimation of cerebral perfusion pressure from arterial blood pressure and transcranial Doppler recordings. In: Miller JD, Teasdale GM, Rowan JO, eds. *Intracranial pressure vi*. Berlin: Springer-Verlag; 1986:226–229.

48. Schmidt EA, Czosnyka M, Gooskens I, et al. Preliminary experience of the estimation of cerebral perfusion pressure using transcranial Doppler ultrasonography. *J Neurol Neurosurg Psychiatry*. 2001;70:198–204.

49. Ragauskas A, Daubaris G, Dziugys A, et al. Innovative non-invasive method for absolute intracranial pressure measurement without calibration. *Acta Neurochir Suppl*. 2005;95:357–361.

50. Bellner J, Romner B, Reinstrup P, et al. Transcranial Doppler sonography pulsatility index (pi) reflects intracranial pressure (icp). *Surg Neurol.* 2004;62:45–51; discussion 51.

51. Kramer DR, Winer JL, Pease BA, et al. Cerebral vasospasm in traumatic brain injury. *Neurology research international.* 2013;2013:415813.

52. Razumovsky A, Tigno T, Hochheimer SM, et al. Cerebral hemodynamic changes after wartime traumatic brain injury. *Acta neurochirurgica. Supplement.* 2013;115:87–90.

53. Rasulo FA, De Peri E, Lavinio A. Transcranial Doppler ultrasonography in intensive care. *European journal of anaesthesiology. Supplement.* 2008;42:167–173.

54. Steiner LA, Balestreri M, Johnston AJ, et al. Sustained moderate reductions in arterial co2 after brain trauma time-course of cerebral blood flow velocity and intracranial pressure. *Intensive Care Med.* 2004;30:2180–2187.

55. Lee JH, Kelly DF, Oertel M, et al. Carbon dioxide reactivity, pressure autoregulation, and metabolic suppression reactivity after head injury: A transcranial Doppler study. *Journal of neurosurgery.* 2001;95:222–232.

56. Bishop CC, Powell S, Rutt D, et al. Transcranial Doppler measurement of middle cerebral artery blood flow velocity: A validation study. *Stroke.* 1986;17:913–915.

57. Obrist WD, Langfitt TW, Jaggi JL, et al. Cerebral blood flow and metabolism in comatose patients with acute head injury. Relationship to intracranial hypertension. *J Neurosurg.* 1984;61:241–253.

58. Marion DW, Bouma GJ. The use of stable xenon-enhanced computed tomographic studies of cerebral blood flow to define changes in cerebral carbon dioxide vasoresponsivity caused by a severe head injury. *Neurosurgery.* 1991;29:869–873.

59. Klingelhofer J, Sander D. Doppler co2 test as an indicator of cerebral vasoreactivity and prognosis in severe intracranial hemorrhages. *Stroke.* 1992;23:962–966.

60. Czosnyka M, Smielewski P, Kirkpatrick P, et al. Monitoring of cerebral autoregulation in head-injured patients. *Stroke.* 1996;27:1829–1834.

61. Lam JM, Hsiang JN, Poon WS. Monitoring of autoregulation using laser Doppler flowmetry in patients with head injury. *J Neurosurg.* 1997;86:438–445.

62. Poon WS, Ng SC, Chan MT, et al. Cerebral blood flow (cbf)-directed management of ventilated head-injured patients. *Acta neurochirurgica. Supplement.* 2005;95:9–11.

63. Lang EW, Diehl RR, Mehdorn HM. Cerebral autoregulation testing after aneurysmal subarachnoid hemorrhage: The phase relationship between arterial blood pressure and cerebral blood flow velocity. *Critical care medicine.* 2001;29:158–163.

64. de Freitas GR, Andre C. Sensitivity of transcranial Doppler for confirming brain death: A prospective study of 270 cases. *Acta Neurol Scand.* 2006;113:426–432.

65. Kuo JR, Chen CF, Chio CC, et al. Time dependent validity in the diagnosis of brain death using transcranial Doppler sonography. *J Neurol Neurosurg Psychiatry.* 2006;77:646–649.

66. Dosemeci L, Dora B, Yilmaz M, et al. Utility of transcranial Doppler ultrasonography for confirmatory diagnosis of brain death: Two sides of the coin. *Transplantation.* 2004;77:71–75.

67. Caplan LR, Mohr JP, Kistler JP, et al. Should thrombolytic therapy be the first-line treatment for acute ischemic stroke? Thrombolysis—not a panacea for ischemic stroke. *The New England journal of medicine.* 1997;337:1309–1310; discussion 1313.

68. Barber PA, Demchuk AM, Hudon ME, et al. Hyperdense sylvian fissure mca "dot" sign: A ct marker of acute ischemia. *Stroke; a journal of cerebral circulation.* 2001;32:84–88.

69. Wildermuth S, Knauth M, Brandt T, et al. Role of CT angiography in patient selection for thrombolytic therapy in acute hemispheric stroke. *Stroke.* 1998;29:935–938.

70. Kenton AR, Martin PJ, Abbott RJ, et al. Comparison of transcranial color-coded sonography and magnetic resonance angiography in acute stroke. *Stroke.* 1997;28:1601–1606.

71. Fieschi C, Argentino C, Lenzi GL, et al. Clinical and instrumental evaluation of patients with ischemic stroke within six hours. *J Neurol Sci* 1989;91:311–322.

72. Zanette EM, Fieschi C, Bozzao L, et al. Comparison of cerebral angiography and transcranial Doppler sonography in acute stroke. *Stroke.* 1989;20:899–903.

73. Kaps M, Link A. Transcranial sonographic monitoring during thrombolytic therapy. *Am J Neuroradiol.* 1998;19:758–760.

74. Razumovsky AY, Gillard JH, Bryan RN, et al. TCD, MRA, and MRI in acute cerebral ischemia. *Acta Neurol Scand.* 1999;99:65–76.

75. Demchuk AM, Christou I, Wein TH, et al. Accuracy and criteria for localizing arterial occlusion with transcranial Doppler. *J Neuroimaging.* 2000;10:1–12.

76. Demchuk AM, Christou I, Wein TH, et al. Specific transcranial Doppler flow findings related to the presence and site of arterial occlusion with transcranial Doppler. *Stroke.* 2000;31:140–146.

77. Moehring MA , Spencer MP. Power M-mode Doppler (PMD) for observing cerebral blood flow and tracking emboli. *Ultrasound Med Biol.* 2002 Jan; 28(1):49–57.

78. Alexandrov AV, Demchuk AM, Burgin WS. Insonation method and diagnostic flow signatures for transcranial power motion (M-mode) Doppler. *J Neuroimaging.* 2002 Jul;12(3):236–244.

79. Barnett SB, Ter Haar GR, Ziskin MC, et l. International recommendations and guidelines for the safe use of diagnostic ultrasound in medicine. *Ultrasound Med Biol.* 2000;26:355–366.

80. Demchuk AM, Wein TH, Felberg RA, et al. Evolution of rapid middle cerebral artery recanalization during intravenous thrombolysis for acute ischemic stroke. *Circulation.* 1999;100:2282–2283.

81. Alexandrov AV, Burgin WS, Demchuk AM, et al. Speed of intracranial clot lysis with intravenous TPA therapy: sonographic classification and short term improvement. *Circulation.* 2001;103: 2897–2902.

82. Christou I, Burgin WS, Alexandrov AV, et al. Arterial status after intravenous TPA therapy for ischemic stroke: a need for further interventions. *Int Angiology.* 2001; Sep20(3):208–213.

83. Kim YS, Garami Z, Mikulik R, et al. and the CLOTBUST Collaborators. Early recanalization rates and clinical outcomes in patients with tandem internal carotid artery/middle cerebral artery occlusion and isolated middle cerebral artery occlusion. *Stroke.* 2005 Apr;36(4):869–871. Epub 2005 Mar 3.

84. Christou I, Alexandrov AV, Burgin WS, et al. Timing of recanalization after tissue plasminogen activator therapy determined by transcranial Doppler correlates with clinical recovery from ischemic stroke. *Stroke.* 2000 Aug;31(8):1812–1816.

85. Alexandrov AV, Burgin WS, Demchuk AM, et al. Speed of intracranial clot lysis with intravenous tissue plasminogen activator therapy: sonographic classification and short-term improvement. *Circulation.* 2001;103:2897–2902.

86. Molina C, Alexandrov AV, Uchino K, et al. for the CLOTBUST Collaborators. MOST: A grading Scale for Ultra-early Prediction of Stroke outcome after thrombolysis. *Stroke.* 2004;35:51–56.

87. Alexandrov AV, Grotta JC. Arterial reocclusion in stroke patients treated with intravenous tissue plasminogen activator. *Neurology.* 2002 Sep 24;59(6):862–862.

88. Rubiera M, Alvarez-Sabin J, Ribo M, et al. Predictors of early arterial reocclusion after tissue plasminogen activator-induced recanalization in acute ischemic stroke. *Stroke.* 2005 Jul;36(7): 1452–1456.

89. Russell D, Madden KP, Clark WM, et al. Detection of arterial emboli using Doppler ultrasound in rabbits. *Stroke.* 1991;22:253–258.

90. Sliwka U, Lingnau L, Stohlmann WD, et al. Prevalence and time course of microembolic signals in patients with acute stroke. *Stroke.* 1997;28:358–363.

91. Valton L, Larrue V, Pavy le Traon A, et al. Microembolic signals and risk of early recurrence inpatients with stroke or transient ischemic attack. *Stroke.* 1998;29:2125–2128.

92. Forteza AM, Babikian VL, Hyde C, et al. Effect of time and cerebrovascular symptoms on the prevalence of microembolic signals in patients with cervical carotid stenosis. *Stroke.* 1996;27: 687–690.

93. Babikian VL, Hyde C, Winter MR. Cerebral microembolism and early recurrent cerebral or retinal ischemic events. *Stroke.* 1997;28:1314–1318.

94. Molloy J, Markus HS. Asymptomatic embolization predicts stroke and TIA risk in patients with carotid artery stenosis. *Stroke.* 1999;30:1440–1443.

95. Gao S, Wong KS, Hansberg T, et al. Microembolic signal predicts recurrent cerebral ischaemic events in acute stroke patients with middle cerebral artery stenosis. *Stroke.* 2004;35:2832–2836.

96. Levi CR, Stork JL, Chambers BR, et al. Dextran reduces embolic signals after carotid endarterectomy. *Ann Neurol.* 2001 Oct;50(4):544–547.

97. Schmidt A, Diederich KW, Scheinert S, et al. Effect of two different neuroprotection systems on microembolization during carotid artery stenting. *J Am Coll Cardiol.* 2004 Nov 16;44(10):1966–1969.

98. Goertler M, Baeumer M, Kross R, et al. Rapid decline of cerebral microemboli of arterial origin after intravenous acetylsalicylic acid. *Stroke.* 1999;30:66–69.

99. Goertler M, Blaser T, Krueger S, et al. Cessation of embolic signals after antithrombotic prevention is related to reduced risk of recurrent arterioembolic transient ischaemic attack and stroke. *J Neurol Neurosurg Psychiatry.* 2002;72:338–342.

100. Markus HS, Droste DW, Kaps M, et al. Dual antiplatelet therapy with clopidogrel and aspirin in symptomatic carotid stenosis evaluated using Doppler embolic signal detection. *Circulation.* 2005;111:2233–2240.

101. Junghans U, Siebler M. Cerebral microembolism is blocked by tirofibran, a selective nonpeptide platelet glycoprotein IIb/IIIa receptor antagonist. *Circulation.* 2003;107:2717–2721.

Continuous EEG Monitoring

Jeremy T. Ragland, MD
Jan Claassen, MD, PhD

INTRODUCTION

Management of critically ill patients relies heavily on continuous cardiac and respiratory monitoring; however, continuous neurologic monitoring is not the standard of care for most intensive care unit (ICU) patients. It can be difficult to monitor neurologic fluctuations in ICU patients that are frequently sedated as well as those with an impaired level of consciousness due to brain injury. Imaging studies like computed tomography (CT), magnetic resonance imaging (MRI), and Doppler ultrasound, provide only a snapshot in time. Continuous monitors are necessary to capture the minute-to-minute physiologic changes that impact patient outcome. Neurophysiological techniques such as electroencephalography (EEG) provide the ability to continuously monitor the brain at the bedside. Medication effects, diurnal variations in level of consciousness or state changes, and structural lesions add to the variability of the data obtained and necessitate contextual interpretation of EEG. Issues of practicality include cost of machinery, maintenance of high-quality recordings, identification of ICU inherent artifacts, nonspecificity of findings, controversial observations, and time-consuming interpretation. However, continuous EEG (cEEG) enables diagnostic and monitoring information that would otherwise not be available.

EEG TECHNIQUES AND USES IN THE INTENSIVE CARE UNIT

Based on the clinical scenario and available resources, different types of EEG monitoring setups can be chosen for the ICU setting. These include spot or single EEG (typically lasting no longer than 30 minutes), serial spot EEGs, continuous surface EEG monitoring with or without quantitative EEG, and EEG with depth electrodes with or without multimodality monitoring. With the advancement in computer technology enabling digital recording and storage of large volumes of EEG data, neurophysiological monitoring has become more rapidly integrated with overall ICU monitoring. The main limitation of obtaining a single EEG recording in the ICU is that it only offers data for a snapshot in time, which may be misleading in a patient with a fluctuating course. Serial EEGs enable the study of evolving patterns and provide a better correlation with the clinical course than a single EEG. Logistical challenges for cEEG monitoring include cost and availability of technicians, purchase of equipment and analytic software, maintenance of electrodes to allow high-quality recordings, and availability of electrophysiologists to interpret the large volume of EEG data (1). cEEG monitoring provides a unique opportunity for the diagnosis and management of various disease states in the ICU. Some of the important applications of EEG monitoring in the ICU setting include: (a) diagnosis and management of status epilepticus (SE), (b) titration of anti-epileptic and sedative medications, (c) detection of nonconvulsive seizures (NCSz) in patients with an unexplained decrease in level of consciousness, (d) detection of periodic electrographic patterns diagnostic of certain disease states such as herpes encephalitis or hepatic encephalopathy, (e) detection of ischemia particularly due to vasospasm after subarachnoid hemorrhage (SAH), (f) prognostication in comatose patients after traumatic brain injury (TBI) or cardiac arrest.

QUANTITATIVE EEG

cEEG generates large amounts of data that are time consuming to interpret. Quantitative EEG (qEEG) tools have been explored that allow rapid screening of long-term recordings. Different quantification methods are available with most commercially available software. Raw EEG data can be quantified after analysis of fast Fourier transform (FFT) of the signal and represented as total power, ratios of power, or spectrograms. These can either be displayed as numbers or graphically as compressed spectral arrays (CSAs), histograms, or as staggered arrays. qEEG graphs can reveal subtle changes over long periods of time that may not be evident when reviewing raw EEG data alone. Parameters for qEEG may include total power, spectral edge frequencies (eg, the frequency below which 50% of the EEG record resides), frequency activity totals (eg, total or percentage alpha power), frequency ratios (eg, alpha-to-delta ratio), amplitude-integrated interval, and brain symmetry index (2,3). Other EEG data reduction display formats include the cerebral function analyzing monitor (CFAM), EEG density modulation, automated analysis of segmented EEG (AAS-EEG), and the bispectral index (BIS) monitor (4,5). For the ICU and acute brain injury, some of these, such as BIS, are highly controversial and may do more harm than good because these reductionist algorithms were developed for different purposes (eg, quantification of anesthetic depth in the operating room). Their validation in the neurologic intensive care unit is lacking. Here the effects of primary and secondary brain injury, medication, recovery from brain injury, and ischemia must be disentangled when interpreting the data.

With the advent of powerful microprocessors, data processing of this type can be performed in real time at the patient's bedside. qEEG analysis is readily available since most manufacturers have integrated it to some extent into their software packages. Importantly, qEEG should never be interpreted in isolation, but should always be seen in the context of the underlying raw EEG. Similar to raw EEG reading, interpretation of qEEG parameters should not be attempted without proper training in electroencephalography. Unfortunately, it is unrealistic to expect 24-hour coverage by an electroencephalographer in all neuro-ICUs. As a result, one approach to data assessment is to have well-trained ICU staff review qEEG parameters and report concerning trends to a remotely stationed electroencephalographer who has access to the correlating raw EEG from a web-based link (6).

AUTOMATED SEIZURE DETECTION

Earlier seizure detection software was primarily based on machine-learning algorithms and analyses of seizures from patients in the epilepsy monitoring units (EMUs) who had ictal activity with a clear onset and offset. Early seizure detection software was primarily based on machine learning algorithms and analyses of seizures from patients in the epilepsy monitoring units (EMUs) who had ictal activity with a clear onset and offset and easy-to-recognize changes in maximum frequency. However, artifacts and nonseizure EEG changes resulted in low sensitivity and specificity for detecting seizures in the ICU. Seizures in the ICU are rarely classical, and borderline-type seizures are frequently encountered, leading to a high false-negative rate (7). Additionally, many patterns frequently encountered in the ICU do not fulfill classic seizure definitions and are characterized by the term "ictal-interictal continuum" (8). Compared to classic seizures, these patterns are often less organized and are without a clear on and off set (1). Much effort has been spent on defining these patterns unequivocally for research purposes (9,10). Recently, automated seizure detection software has used ICU datasets to create algorithms and anecdotally have increased the specificity and sensitivity for ICU seizure detection. Again, none of these algorithms are accurate enough to replace reading of the raw EEG. Given the variability of qEEG findings encountered following acute brain injury, there is some doubt that this will ever be accomplished. Seizure detection programs make use of specialized EEG processing software that can be used to screen large amounts of continuously recorded EEG data. The programs then mark sections containing activity suspicious for seizures. Based on an FFT analysis of the EEG, CSA graphs can be generated to determine the occurrence of subclincial seizures. Once the "CSA signature" of a seizure in an individual patient has been determined, it can be used to quickly screen a 24-hour recording and quantify the frequency of seizures (11).

DEPTH AND SURFACE EEG RECORDING WITH MULTIMODALITY MONITORING

Invasive multimodality brain monitoring is increasingly used to monitor comatose patients with severe brain injury to detect evolving injury earlier, prevent secondary brain injury, and individualize treatment goals in the aftermath of acute brain injury (eg, prevention of metabolic crisis). A number of different devices are available to measure and track either upstream effectors or downstream indicators of neuronal health, including neuronal activity, brain metabolism, brain tissue oxygenation, and perfusion (12). Surface and depth EEG monitoring may become an integral part of multimodality monitoring, but few studies have investigated this to date (13–17).

Preliminary studies suggest that a mini depth electrode inserted into the cortex may augment data obtained from surface EEG. Depth electrode readings may improve the signal-to-noise ratio of EEG (ie, shivering obliterating surface recordings), clarify suspicious but not clearly epileptiform patterns (ie, rhythmic slowing without clear evolution), detect seizures not seen on the surface, and detect changes that indicate secondary complications (eg, ischemia) (15). However, the significance of depth-only findings is currently unclear and should not lead to management changes without additional data to corroborate the impression (Figure 3.1; 18).

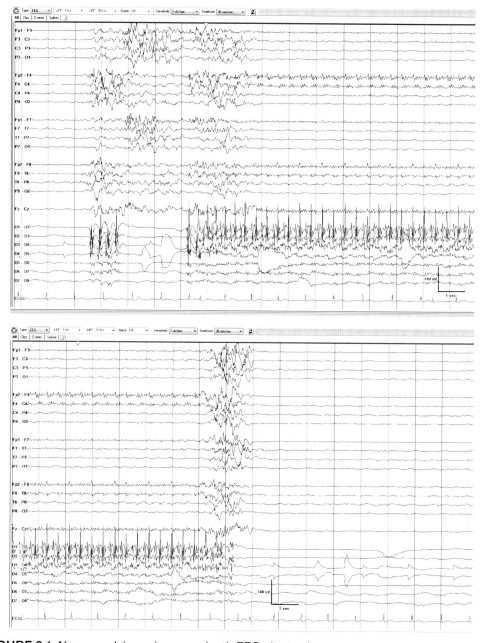

FIGURE 3.1 Nonconvulsive seizure on depth EEG electrode.

This continuous EEG reveals a train of low voltage 12–14 Hz rhythmic beta activity in the right frontal region between higher voltage diffuse bursts. A right frontal depth electrode (represented by leads D1–D8) reveals an ictal correlate composed of higher voltage 7–8 Hz spike and wave discharges.

EEG APPLICATIONS

Subclinical Seizures and Status Epilepticus

Acute seizures and (SE) are common in all types of acute brain injury and are not restricted to patients with epilepsy. Almost all seizures in the ICU setting are nonconvulsive and not detectable unless EEG monitoring is employed. Patients with NCSz may occasionally demonstrate very subtle clinical signs of seizure. These signs include face and limb myoclonus, nystagmus, eye deviation, pupillary abnormalities (including hippus), and autonomic instability (19–24). However, none of these clinical manifestations is specific for NCSz, and cEEG is usually necessary to confirm or refute the diagnosis of NCSz (Figure 3.2). The underlying etiologies for convulsive SE and nonconvulsive SE (NCSE) may be similar. These include structural lesions, infections, metabolic derangements, toxins, withdrawal, and epilepsy, all of which are common diagnoses in the critically ill patient (25).

NCSz are seen in 48% and NCSE in 14% of patients following control of convulsions in generalized convulsive status epilepticus (GCSE) (26). NCSE can be found in 8% of medical ICU patients who are devoid of any clinical signs of seizure activity and have no history of neurologic disease (24,27). In neurologic ICUs, up to 34% of comatose patients have NCSz, and 76% of them have NCSE (28). Patients on continuous IV antiepileptic drugs (AEDs) for the treatment of refractory SE should always be monitored with cEEG, since subclinical seizures may occur in more than half of patients during treatment. The majority of these patients will also have subclinical seizures after discontinuation of therapy (11,29). Therefore, cEEG should be performed on any patient who does not quickly regain consciousness after a convulsive seizure to detect ongoing seizure activity. This includes patients who are sedated and/or paralyzed during the treatment of SE in whom level of consciousness cannot be adequately assessed. NCSE in the ICU setting is associated with high morbidity and mortality (24,30–32).

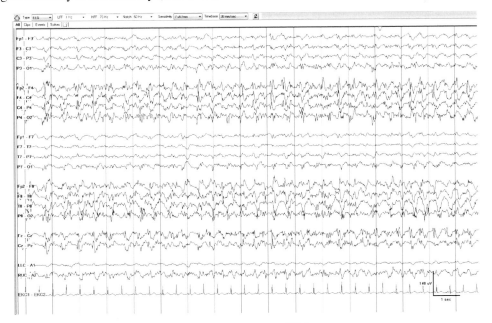

FIGURE 3.2 Nonconvulsive seizure (NCSz) on scalp EEG.

This continuous EEG reveals a right hemispheric seizure.

Duration of Monitoring

There are no prospective studies that have evaluated different durations of cEEG monitoring in patients with SE. A retrospective analysis of electrographic data obtained from patients who had a depressed level of consciousness from an undetermined cause revealed that 20% of patients did not have their first seizure until after 24 hours of monitoring and 13% did not have their first seizure until more than 48 hours of monitoring (23). For noncomatose patients, most seizure activity was detected early (23). Recently published guidelines recommend that delays in initiating cEEG monitoring should be minimized as the cumulative duration of SE affects neurologic outcomes and mortality (29,33). These guidelines further recommend at least 48 hours of monitoring for comatose patients with acute brain injury and at least 24 hours for those that are not comatose.

EEG Findings

Efforts are underway to standardize (at least for research purposes) definitions of ictal and interictal EEG patterns (10). There has been much controversy regarding the interpretation and therapeutic implications of treating periodic epileptiform discharges that do not meet formal seizure criteria (8,34,35). Periodic lateralized epileptiform discharges (PLEDs) may be both ictal and interictal and at times may be an indicator of encephalopathy (36,37). Supplemental information regarding their ictal/interictal nature can be determined by using serial EEG data (38,39), focal hyperperfusion single-photon-emission computed tomography (40), and increased metabolism on fluorodeoxyglucose positron emission tomography (41). Periodic epileptiform discharges may represent ictal activity in the comatose patient if they are associated with some type of evolution in frequency, amplitude, and space. Additional testing with a benzodiazepine trial, imaging studies, serum markers, or invasive brain monitoring may guide the physician in managing patients with these EEG findings (Figure 3.3; 42).

Metabolic and Infectious Encephalopathies

Critically ill patients are susceptible to many toxic, metabolic, and electrolyte imbalances that may cause both changes in mental status and seizures. Over a 2-year period, 12.3% of 1,758 patients admitted to the medical ICU experienced some type of neurologic complications. Among these, metabolic encephalopathy was the most common complication, followed by seizures (28%), which usually occurred in the setting of metabolic derangement (43). Reasons include, but are not limited to, hypo- and hyperglycemia, hyponatremia, hypocalcemia, drug intoxication or withdrawal, uremia, liver dysfunction, hypertensive encephalopathy, and sepsis. The incidence of NCSz can vary from 5% to 22% (25). In neurologic and medical ICU patients, sepsis and acute renal failure may be associated with electrographic seizures (24,25). While certain periodic discharges are more closely related to systemic metabolic abnormalities, such as triphasic waves in hepatic encephalopathy, the significance of others such as periodic lateralized epileptiform discharges PLEDs is controversial.

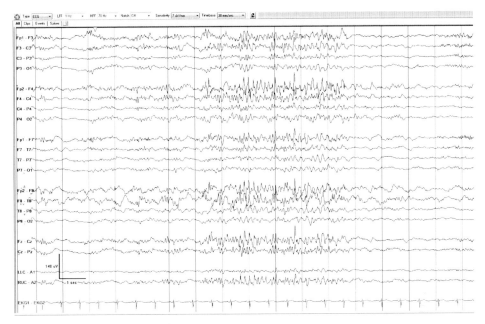

FIGURE 3.3 Ictal-interictal continuum.

The cEEG reveals a focal 6-second burst of sharply contoured theta discharges predominantly seen in the right frontotemporal region. While not definitely ictal, this finding is highly epileptogenic and lies on the ictal-interictal continuum.

Traumatic Brain Injury

Between 15% and 22% of patients with moderate to severe TBI can have convulsive seizures. However, the incidence of NCSz is less well studied (44–46). The exact relationship between seizures and outcome is unclear, but some studies have shown that early posttraumatic seizures are an independent risk factor for poor outcome in adults (47).

EEG monitoring in TBI patients may be used to monitor clinical course, titration of sedative medications, and for diagnosing posttraumatic complications such as seizures. The goal remains to individualize therapeutic approaches in order to detect secondary brain injury as early as possible and to prevent further damage such as focal ischemia.

To manage intracranial pressure, high-dose barbiturates, benzodiazepines, or propofol infusions may be needed in TBI patients. While the ICP monitor is the primary tool used to guide therapy when managing elevated ICP, EEG may be used as a supplement when the goal of therapy is to induce burst suppression.

A number of EEG findings are associated with outcome following acute brain injury. These include seizures, periodic discharges, lack of sleep architecture, and EEG reactivity (48). A quantitative EEG monitoring study in TBI patients used changes in the EEG variability approach to predict outcome (49). Data reduction was achieved by focusing on the percentage of alpha-frequencies (PA) at multiple electrodes and the determination of its variability (PAV) over time. A low PAV and especially a decrease in PAV over time strongly correlated with a fatal outcome, especially in patients with low Glascow coma scores. PAV values obtained during the initial 3 days after injury were significantly associated with outcome, independent of clinical and radiological parameters.

Outcome prediction in TBI patients may utilize EEG background attenuation and low-amplitude events in the EEG by quantification of periods of EEG suppression to derive the EEG silence ratio (ESR) (50). In a study of 32 TBI patients, the authors showed that outcome at 6 months was closely related to ESR values obtained within the first 4 days following head injury. However, this method is limited by artificial increases of the ESR related to sedation.

Subarachnoid Hemorrhage

In patients with SAH, seizures may occur at the time of the hemorrhage, in the hospital, and long after discharge. Underlying mechanisms differ, but all are associated with worse outcome. In a series of 108 SAH patients who underwent cEEG for altered mental status or suspicion of seizures, 19% had seizures (51). Most of these seizures were NCSz, and 70% of patients with seizures had NCSE. Another study analyzed intracortical EEG and multimodality physiology in 48 comatose patients following SAH. Intracortical seizures were seen in 38% of patients, while only 8% had surface seizures. The authors found that functional outcome was very poor for patients with severe background attenuation, while outcome was best in patients without severe attenuation or seizures (77% vs 0% dead or severely disabled, respectively). Patients with seizures independent of background EEG had intermediate outcome. Those with only intracortical seizures had worse outcomes compared to those with intracortical and scalp seizures (50% vs 25% dead or severely disabled, respectively (Figure 3.4; 52). cEEG monitoring provides independent prognostic information in patients with poor-grade SAH, even after controlling for clinical and radiological findings. Unfavorable findings include periodic epileptiform discharges, electrographic SE, and the absence of sleep architecture (53).

Detection of Vasospasm

In the neuro ICU setting, quantitative analysis of cEEG has been used to detect delayed cerebral ischemia (DCI) due to vasospasm in SAH patients (54–56). There is still

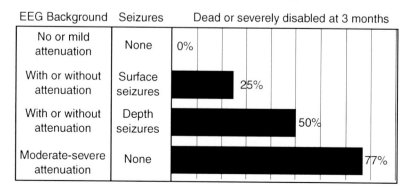

FIGURE 3.4 Three-month functional outcome after SAH stratified by EEG background activity and presence of intracortical or surface seizures.

controversy over the qEEG parameter that best correlates with clinically significant ischemia, but most authors agree that a ratio of fast over slow activity (eg, alpha-to-delta ratio, or relative alpha variability) is the most practical approach (51,54,57). A number of qEEG parameters have been shown to correlate with DCI or angiographic vasospasm: trend analysis of total power (1–30 Hz; 56), variability of relative alpha (6–14 Hz/1–20 Hz; 54), and poststimulation alpha-delta ratio (PSADR, 8–13 Hz/1–4 Hz; 55). In a retrospective study of 34 poor-grade SAH patients (Hunt-Hess Grades 4 and 5) monitored from postoperative days 2 to 14, it was found that a reduction in the poststimulation ratio of alpha and delta frequency power of greater than 10% relative to baseline in six consecutive epochs of qEEG was 100% sensitive and 76% specific for DCI. A reduction of greater than 50% in a single epoch was 89% sensitive and 84% specific for diagnosing DCI (55). These qEEG parameters may detect changes up to 2 days prior to clinical deterioration. Importantly, all of these studies found that focal ischemia sometimes resulted in global or bilateral changes in the EEG, and EEG changes may precede clinical deterioration by several days (54). Rathakrishnan et al studied a variation of previously described qEEG parameters termed composite alpha index (CAI). CAI measures relative alpha power and variability in the anterior brain quadrants and can be graphically displayed (58). Twelve patients with DCI were studied by trending the daily mean alpha power against the modulation of treatment and clinical evolution. Sensitivity of predicting clinical deterioration with cEEG improved from 40% to 67%. In three patients, cEEG was predictive greater than 24 hours prior to clinical change. Tracking the daily mean alpha power accurately identified DCI recurrence and poor responders to first-line therapy at preclinical stages. In a small feasibility study, it was reported that intracortical EEG was a promising tool for detecting ischemia from vasospasm in poor-grade SAH patients and may be superior to scalp EEG (Figure 3.5; 18).

It has long been known that infarction may result in polymorphic delta, loss of fast activity and sleep spindles, and focal attenuation. These EEG findings have been shown to reflect abnormal cerebral blood flow (CBF) and cerebral metabolic rate of oxygen as demonstrated by positron emission tomography(PET) and Xenon-CT-CBF imaging (59,60). EEG is very sensitive for ischemia and usually demonstrates changes at the time of reversible neuronal dysfunction (CBF 25–30 mL/100 g/min) (61). EEG is also very sensitive for recovery and may demonstrate recovery of brain function from reperfusion earlier than the clinical exam (62).

Intracerebral Hemorrhage

Intracerebral hemorrhage (ICH) is associated with a 3% to 19% rate of in-hospital convulsive seizures (63–67). In two studies using cEEG, 18% to 21% of patients with ICH were shown to have NCSz (63,68). Continuous EEG findings may also predict outcome after ICH. One study found that NCSz were associated with increased midline shift and were associated with a trend toward worse outcomes, after controlling for hemorrhage size (68). In a subsequent study of ICH patients, NCSz were associated with expansion of hemorrhage volume and mass effect, and a trend toward worse outcomes (63). In addition, periodic epileptiform discharges (PEDs) were an independent predictor of poor outcome.

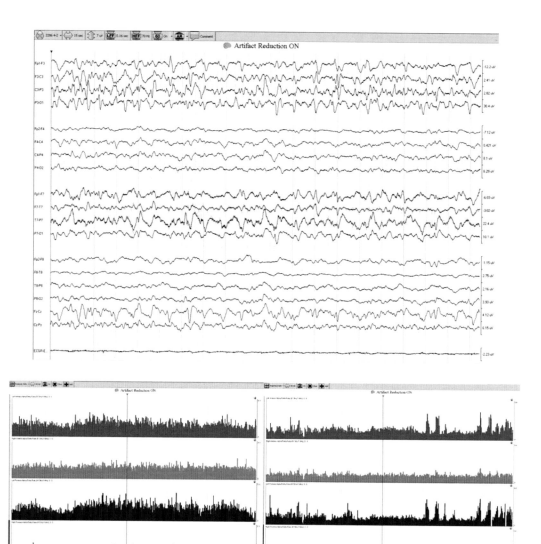

FIGURE 3.5 Detection of ischemia.

Panel A shows the surface EEG of a patient with SAH due to right middle cerebral artery (MCA) aneurysm rupture. The recording was obtained during a period of right MCA vasospasm and reveals moderate-to-diffuse slowing more prominent over the right hemisphere. Panel B shows the alpha-to-delta (ADR) ratio in the same patient. The left portion shows ADR prior to vasospasm, and the right panel shows the ADR during vasospasm. Note that the ADR decreases in the setting of vasospasm particularly on the right side. Tracings from top to bottom are left anterior, right anterior, left posterior, and right posterior. (Figures courtesy of Brandon Foreman, MD.)

Ischemic Stroke

EEG will not replace imaging in the diagnosis of ischemic stroke, as imaging is more readily available and more specific for detection of stroke. However, EEG can be used to monitor for response to treatment (eg, augmentation of blood pressure) in ischemic stroke, and monitoring over time may lead to early seizure diagnosis.

Seizure Detection

A population-based cEEG study in 177 patients with ischemic stroke reported a 7% incidence of seizures (more than 70% NCSz) in the acute (within 24 hours) phase, and hospital-based studies have reported rates of acute clinical seizures following ischemic stroke ranging from 2% to 9% (64,65,67). Several studies have shown that acute clinical seizures are associated with increased mortality in patients with ischemic stroke (64,65,69,70). In a prospective study of 232 patients, EEG recording was performed within 24 hours from hospitalization and continued for 1 week. Fifteen patients (6.5%) had early seizures within 24 hours; 10 of these patients had focal SE with or without secondary generalization. EEG revealed sporadic epileptiform focal abnormalities in 10% and PLEDs in 6%. SE was recorded in 71.4% of patients with PLEDs. The authors concluded that seizures are not frequent on the acute phase of ischemic stroke. However, when present, they often occur as focal SE at onset (71).

Prognosis Following Ischemic Stroke

In a prospective study, 25 patients underwent cEEG monitoring after malignant middle cerebral artery (MCA) territory infarction. In these patients, the absence of delta activity and the presence of theta and fast beta frequencies within the focus of the infarct predicted a benign course ($P < .05$). Diffuse generalized slowing and slow delta activity in the ischemic hemisphere predicted a malignant course (72). A decrease in CPP is associated with reduction in faster EEG activity (73). Rapid improvements in background EEG activity have been observed when cerebral perfusion pressure (CPP) and CBF increase following mannitol or hemodilution therapy (74,75).

Post–Cardiac Arrest

In patients with hypoxic-ischemic encephalopathy after cardiac arrest, the presence of seizures may have important prognostic value and also be a potential contributor to decreased mental status (76). As hypothermia after cardiac arrest for neuro-protection becomes more widely implemented, cEEG may become an important tool for identifying NCSz, especially during rewarming (77). Myoclonic and nonconvulsive SE is common in comatose post–cardiac arrest patients undergoing therapeutic hypothermia, and most seizures occur within the first 8 hours of cEEG recording and within the first 12 hours after resuscitation from cardiac arrest (76,78,79). Outcomes are poor in those who experience NCSE and convulsive SE (76,78,79).

In patients treated with hypothermia, EEG monitoring during the first 24 hours after resuscitation can contribute to the prediction of both good and poor neurologic outcome. Continuous patterns within 12 hours predicted good outcome. Isoelectric or low-voltage EEGs after 24 hours predicted poor outcome with a sensitivity almost two times larger than bilateral absent somatosensory evoked potential responses (80). EEG reactivity significantly improved prognostication in patients treated with therapeutic hypothermia following cardiac arrest (81).

In a study of 192 (103 hypothermic, 89 nonhypothermic) patients post–cardiac arrest, myoclonic SE was invariably associated with death ($P = .0002$). Malignant EEG patterns and global cerebral edema on head CT were associated with death in both populations ($P < .001$) (82). In a study of 47 conscious survivors of cardiac arrest (27 in the hypothermia group and 18 in normothermia group), quantitative electroencephalography (qEEG), and auditory P300 event-related potentials were studied on 42 patients. No differences were found in any of the cognitive functions between the two groups at 3-month follow-up. Sixty-seven percent of patients in hypothermia and 44% patients in normothermia group were cognitively intact or had only very mild impairment. Severe cognitive deficits were found in 15% and 28% of patients, respectively. All qEEG parameters were better in the hypothermia-treated group, but the differences did not reach statistical significance. The amplitude of P300 potential was significantly higher in hypothermia-treated group. This study concluded that the use of therapeutic hypothermia was not associated with cognitive decline or neurophysiological deficits after out-of-hospital cardiac arrest (83).

Despite these data, the prognostic certainty of EEG findings must be questioned, as there is anecdotal evidence of good outcomes even in patients with SE after cardiac arrest.

Postoperative Patients

Seizures can occur in any postoperative setting where there is an acute neurologic injury, a high risk of metabolic derangement, or neurotoxicity. Postoperative cEEG monitoring may be indicated in patients undergoing surgery for supratentorial lesions or patients who had pre-existing epilepsy (84,85). Other high-risk groups include patients undergoing cardiac surgery or solid organ transplants (86–88). However, the incidence of NCSz and NCSE in these patients has not been studied systematically.

REFERENCES

1. Hirsch LJ, Claassen J. The current state of treatment of status epilepticus. *Current Neurology and Neuroscience Reports.* 2002;2:345–356.
2. Suzuki A, Mori N, Hadeishi H, et al. Computerized monitoring system in neurosurgical intensive care. *Journal of Neuroscience Methods.* 1988;26:133–139.
3. Agarwal R, Gotman J, Flanagan D, et al. Automatic EEG analysis during long-term monitoring in the ICU. *Electroencephalogr Clin Neurophysiol.* 1998;107:44–58.
4. Newton DE. Electrophysiological monitoring of general intensive care patients. *Intensive Care Med.* 1999;25:350–352.
5. Maynard DE, Jenkinson JL. The cerebral function analysing monitor. Initial clinical experience, application and further development. *Anaesthesia.* 1984;39:678–690.
6. Scheuer ML, Wilson SB. Data analysis for continuous EEG monitoring in the ICU: seeing the forest and the trees. *J Clin Neurophysiol.* 2004;21:353–378.
7. Tasker RC, Boyd SG, Harden A, et al. The cerebral function analysing monitor in paediatric medical intensive care: applications and limitations. *Intensive Care Medicine.* 1990;16:60–68.
8. Pohlmann-Eden B, Hoch DB, Cochius JI, et al. Periodic lateralized epileptiform discharges— a critical review. *Journal of Clinical Neurophysiology: Official Publication of the American Electroencephalographic Society.* 1996;13:519–530.
9. Albers D CJ, Schmidt JM, Hripcsak G. (in press). A methodology for detecting and exploring non-convulsive seizures in patients with SAH. *IEICE* 2013.
10. Hirsch LJ, LaRoche SM, Gaspard N, et al. American Clinical Neurophysiology Society's Standardized Critical Care EEG Terminology: 2012 version. *Journal of Clinical Neurophysiology: Official Publication of the American Electroencephalographic Society.* 2013;30:1–27.
11. Claassen J, Baeumer T, Hansen HC. [Continuous EEG for monitoring on the neurological intensive care unit. New applications and uses for therapeutic decision making]. *Nervenarzt.* 2000;71:813–821.
12. Wartenberg KE, Schmidt JM, Mayer SA. Multimodality monitoring in neurocritical care. *Crit Care Clin.* 2007;23:507–538.

13. Miller CM, Vespa PM, McArthur DL, et al. Frameless stereotactic aspiration and thrombolysis of deep intracerebral hemorrhage is associated with reduced levels of extracellular cerebral glutamate and unchanged lactate pyruvate ratios. *Neurocritical Care.* 2007;6:22–29.

14. Vespa P, Prins M, Ronne-Engstrom E, et al. Increase in extracellular glutamate caused by reduced cerebral perfusion pressure and seizures after human traumatic brain injury: a microdialysis study. *Journal of Neurosurgery.* 1998;89:971–982.

15. Waziri A, Claassen J, Stuart RM, et al. Intracortical electroencephalography in acute brain injury. *Annals of Neurology.* 2009;66:366–377.

16. Claassen J PA, Albers D, Kleinberg S, et al. Nonconvulsive seizures after subarachnoid hemorrhage: multimodality detection and outcomes. *Annals of Neurology* (in press).

17. Nangunoori R, Maloney-Wilensky E, Stiefel M, et al. Brain tissue oxygen-based therapy and outcome after severe traumatic brain injury: a systematic literature review. *Neurocritical Care.* 2012;17: 131–138.

18. Stuart RM, Waziri A, Weintraub D, et al. Intracortical EEG for the detection of vasospasm in patients with poor-grade subarachnoid hemorrhage. *Neurocrit Care.* 2010;13:355–358.

19. Jirsch J, Hirsch LJ. Nonconvulsive seizures: developing a rational approach to the diagnosis and management in the critically ill population. *Clin Neurophysiol.* 2007;118:1660–1670.

20. Husain AM, Horn GJ, Jacobson MP. Non-convulsive status epilepticus: usefulness of clinical features in selecting patients for urgent EEG. *J Neurol Neurosurg Psychiatry.* 2003;74:189–191.

21. Kaplan PW. Behavioral Manifestations of Nonconvulsive Status Epilepticus. *Epilepsy Behav.* 2002;3:122–139.

22. Lowenstein DH, Aminoff MJ. Clinical and EEG features of status epilepticus in comatose patients. *Neurology.* 1992;42:100–104.

23. Claassen J, Mayer SA, Kowalski RG, et al. Detection of electrographic seizures with continuous EEG monitoring in critically ill patients. *Neurology.* 2004;62:1743–1748.

24. Oddo M, Carrera E, Claassen J, et al. Continuous electroencephalography in the medical intensive care unit. *Crit Care Med.* 2009;37:2051–2056.

25. Abou Khaled KJ, Hirsch LJ. Advances in the management of seizures and status epilepticus in critically ill patients. *Crit Care Clin.* 2006;22:637–659; abstract viii.

26. DeLorenzo RJ, Waterhouse EJ, Towne AR, et al. Persistent nonconvulsive status epilepticus after the control of convulsive status epilepticus. *Epilepsia.* 1998;39:833–840.

27. Towne AR, Waterhouse EJ, Boggs JG, et al. Prevalence of nonconvulsive status epilepticus in comatose patients. *Neurology.* 2000;54:340–345.

28. Jordan KG. Neurophysiologic monitoring in the neuroscience intensive care unit. *Neurol Clin.* 1995;13:579–626.

29. Brophy GM, Bell R, Claassen J, et al. Guidelines for the evaluation and management of status epilepticus. *Neurocritical Care.* 2012;17:3–23.

30. Young GB, Jordan KG, Doig GS. An assessment of nonconvulsive seizures in the intensive care unit using continuous EEG monitoring: an investigation of variables associated with mortality. *Neurology.* 1996;47:83–89.

31. Krumholz A, Sung GY, Fisher RS, et al. Complex partial status epilepticus accompanied by serious morbidity and mortality. *Neurology.* 1995;45:1499–1504.

32. Litt B, Wityk RJ, Hertz SH, et al. Nonconvulsive status epilepticus in the critically ill elderly. *Epilepsia.* 1998;39:1194–1202.

33. Claassen J, Taccone FS, Horn P, et al. Recommendations on the use of EEG monitoring in critically ill patients: consensus statement from the neurointensive care section of the ESICM. *Intensive Care Med.* 2013;39:1337–1351.

34. Treiman DM. Electroclinical features of status epilepticus. *Journal of Clinical Neurophysiology: Official Publication of the American Electroencephalographic Society.* 1995;12:343–362.

35. Husain AM, Mebust KA, Radtke RA. Generalized periodic epileptiform discharges: etiologies, relationship to status epilepticus, and prognosis. *Journal of Clinical Neurophysiology: Official Publication of the American Electroencephalographic Society.* 1999;16:51–58.

36. Kaplan PW. Assessing the outcomes in patients with nonconvulsive status epilepticus: nonconvulsive status epilepticus is underdiagnosed, potentially overtreated, and confounded by comorbidity. *J Clin Neurophysiol.* 1999;16:341–353.

37. Niedermeyer E, Ribeiro M. Considerations of nonconvulsive status epilepticus. *Clinical EEG.* 2000;31:192–195.

38. Garzon E, Fernandes RM, Sakamoto AC. Serial EEG during human status epilepticus: evidence for PLED as an ictal pattern. *Neurology.* 2001;57:1175–1183.

39. Treiman DM, Walton NY, Kendrick C. A progressive sequence of electroencephalographic changes during generalized convulsive status epilepticus. *Epilepsy Research.* 1990;5:49–60.

40. Assal F, Papazyan JP, Slosman DO, et al. SPECT in periodic lateralized epileptiform discharges (PLEDs): a form of partial status epilepticus? *Seizure.* 2001;10:260–265.

41. Handforth A, Cheng JT, Mandelkern MA, et al. Markedly increased mesiotemporal lobe metabolism in a case with PLEDs: further evidence that PLEDs are a manifestation of partial status epilepticus. *Epilepsia.* 1994;35:876–881.

42. Claassen J. How I treat patients with EEG patterns on the ictal-interictal continuum in the neuro ICU. *Neurocrit Care.* 2009;11:437–444.

43. Bleck TP, Smith MC, Pierre-Louis SJ, et al. Neurologic complications of critical medical illness. *Crit Care Med.* 1993;21:98–103.

44. Annegers JF, Grabow JD, Groover RV, et al. Seizures after head trauma: a population study. *Neurology.* 1980;30:683–689.

45. Temkin NR, Dikmen SS, Wilensky AJ, et al. A randomized, double-blind study of phenytoin for the prevention of post-traumatic seizures. *N Engl J Med.* 1990;323:497–502.

46. Vespa P. Continuous EEG monitoring for the detection of seizures in traumatic brain injury, infarction, and intracerebral hemorrhage: "to detect and protect." *J Clin Neurophysiol.* 2005;22:99–106.

47. Wang HC, Chang WN, Chang HW, et al. Factors predictive of outcome in posttraumatic seizures. *J Trauma.* 2008;64:883–888.

48. Rae-Grant AD, Barbour PJ, Reed J. Development of a novel EEG rating scale for head injury using dichotomous variables. *Electroencephalography and Slinical Neurophysiology.* 1991;79:349–357.

49. Vespa PM, Boscardin WJ, Hovda DA, et al. Early and persistent impaired percent alpha variability on continuous electroencephalography monitoring as predictive of poor outcome after traumatic brain injury. *Journal of Neurosurgery.* 2002;97:84–92.

50. Theilen HJ, Ragaller M, Tscho U, et al. Electroencephalogram silence ratio for early outcome prognosis in severe head trauma. *Crit Care Med.* 2000;28:3522–3529.

51. Friedman D, Claassen J, Hirsch LJ. Continuous electroencephalogram monitoring in the intensive care unit. *Anesth Analg.* 2009;109:506–523.

52. Claassen J, Perotte A, Albers D, et al. Nonconvulsive Seizures after Subarachnoid Hemorrhage: Multimodal Detection and Outcomes. *Ann Neurol.* 2013;74:53–64.

53. Claassen J, Hirsch LJ, Frontera JA, et al. Prognostic significance of continuous EEG monitoring in patients with poor-grade subarachnoid hemorrhage. *Neurocritical Care.* 2006;4:103–112.

54. Vespa PM, Nuwer MR, Juhasz C, et al. Early detection of vasospasm after acute subarachnoid hemorrhage using continuous EEG ICU monitoring. *Electroencephalography and Clinical Neurophysiology.* 1997;103:607–615.

55. Claassen J, Hirsch LJ, Kreiter KT, et al. Quantitative continuous EEG for detecting delayed cerebral ischemia in patients with poor-grade subarachnoid hemorrhage. *Clinical Neurophysiology: Official Journal of the International Federation of Clinical Neurophysiology.* 2004;115:2699–2710.

56. Labar DR, Fisch BJ, Pedley TA, et al. Quantitative EEG monitoring for patients with subarachnoid hemorrhage. *Electroencephalogr Clin Neurophysiol.* 1991;78:325–332.

57. Foreman B, Claassen J. Quantitative EEG for the detection of brain ischemia. *Crit Care.* 2012;16:216.

58. Rathakrishnan R, Gotman J, Dubeau F, et al. Using continuous electroencephalography in the management of delayed cerebral ischemia following subarachnoid hemorrhage. *Neurocritical Care.* 2011;14:152–161.

59. Nagata K, Tagawa K, Hiroi S, et al. Electroencephalographic correlates of blood flow and oxygen metabolism provided by positron emission tomography in patients with cerebral infarction. *Electroencephalography and Clinical Neurophysiology.* 1989;72:16–30.

60. Tolonen U, Sulg IA. Comparison of quantitative EEG parameters from four different analysis techniques in evaluation of relationships between EEG and CBF in brain infarction. *Electroencephalography and Clinical Neurophysiology.* 1981;51:177–185.

61. Astrup J, Siesjo BK, Symon L. Thresholds in cerebral ischemia—the ischemic penumbra. *Stroke.* 1981;12:723–725.

62. Jordan KG. Emergency EEG and continuous EEG monitoring in acute ischemic stroke. *J Clin Neurophysiol*. 2004;21:341–52.

63. Claassen J, Jette N, Chum F, et al. Electrographic seizures and periodic discharges after intracerebral hemorrhage. *Neurology*. 2007;69:1356–1365.

64. Bladin CF, Alexandrov AV, Bellavance A, et al. Seizures after stroke: a prospective multicenter study. *Arch Neurol*. 2000;57:1617–1622.

65. Arboix A. [Epileptic crisis and cerebral vascular disease]. *Rev Clin Esp*. 1997;197:346–350.

66. Faught E, Peters D, Bartolucci A, et al. Seizures after primary intracerebral hemorrhage. *Neurology*. 1989;39:1089–1093.

67. Szaflarski JP, Rackley AY, Kleindorfer DO, et al. Incidence of seizures in the acute phase of stroke: a population-based study. *Epilepsia*. 2008;49:974–981.

68. Vespa PM, O'Phelan K, Shah M, et al. Acute seizures after intracerebral hemorrhage: a factor in progressive midline shift and outcome. *Neurology*. 2003;60:1441–1446.

69. Arboix A, Comes E, Massons J, et al. Relevance of early seizures for in-hospital mortality in acute cerebrovascular disease. *Neurology*. 1996;47:1429–1435.

70. Vernino S, Brown RD, Jr., Sejvar JJ, et al. Cause-specific mortality after first cerebral infarction: a population-based study. *Stroke*. 2003;34:1828–1832.

71. Mecarelli O, Pro S, Randi F, et al. EEG patterns and epileptic seizures in acute phase stroke. *Cerebrovasc Dis*. 2011;31:191–198.

72. Burghaus L, Hilker R, Dohmen C, et al. Early electroencephalography in acute ischemic stroke: prediction of a malignant course? *Clinical Neurology and Neurosurgery*. 2007;109:45–49.

73. Diedler J, Sykora M, Bast T, et al. Quantitative EEG correlates of low cerebral perfusion in severe stroke. *Neurocritical Care*. 2009;11:210–216.

74. Huang Z, Dong W, Yan Y, et al. Effects of intravenous mannitol on EEG recordings in stroke patients. *Clinical Neurophysiology: Official Journal of the International Federation of Clinical Neurophysiology*. 2002;113:446–453.

75. Wood JH, Polyzoidis KS, Epstein CM, et al. Quantitative EEG alterations after isovolemic-hemodilutional augmentation of cerebral perfusion in stroke patients. *Neurology*. 1984;34:764–768.

76. Rossetti AO, Logroscino G, Liaudet L, et al. Status epilepticus: an independent outcome predictor after cerebral anoxia. *Neurology*. 2007;69:255–260.

77. Hovland A, Nielsen EW, Kluver J, et al. EEG should be performed during induced hypothermia. *Resuscitation*. 2006;68:143–146.

78. Legriel S, Bruneel F, Sediri H, et al. Early EEG monitoring for detecting postanoxic status epilepticus during therapeutic hypothermia: a pilot study. *Neurocritical care*. 2009;11:338–344.

79. Rittenberger JC, Popescu A, Brenner RP, et al. Frequency and timing of nonconvulsive status epilepticus in comatose post-cardiac arrest subjects treated with hypothermia. *Neurocritical care*. 2012;16:114–122.

80. Cloostermans MC, van Meulen FB, Eertman CJ, et al. Continuous electroencephalography monitoring for early prediction of neurological outcome in postanoxic patients after cardiac arrest: a prospective cohort study. *Crit Care Med*. 2012;40:2867–2875.

81. Rossetti AO, Oddo M, Logroscino G, Kaplan PW. Prognostication after cardiac arrest and hypothermia: a prospective study. *Annals of Neurology*. 2010;67:301–307.

82. Fugate JE, Wijdicks EF, Mandrekar J, et al. Predictors of neurologic outcome in hypothermia after cardiac arrest. *Annals of Neurology*. 2010;68:907–914.

83. Tiainen M, Poutiainen E, Kovala T, et al. Cognitive and neurophysiological outcome of cardiac arrest survivors treated with therapeutic hypothermia. *Stroke*. 2007;38:2303–2308.

84. Matthew E, Sherwin AL, Welner SA, et al. Seizures following intracranial surgery: incidence in the first post-operative week. *Can J Neurol Sci*. 1980;7:285–290.

85. Foy PM, Copeland GP, Shaw MD. The incidence of postoperative seizures. *Acta Neurochir (Wien)*. 1981;55:253–264.

86. Llinas R, Barbut D, Caplan LR. Neurologic complications of cardiac surgery. *Prog Cardiovasc Dis*. 2000;43:101–112.

87. Wijdicks EF, Plevak DJ, Wiesner RH, et al. Causes and outcome of seizures in liver transplant recipients. *Neurology*. 1996;47:1523–1525.

88. Vaughn BV, Ali, II, Olivier KN, et al. Seizures in lung transplant recipients. *Epilepsia,*. 1996;37:1175–1179.

Cerebral Oxygenation

Michel T. Torbey, MD
Chad M. Miller, MD

INTRODUCTION

Monitoring of the brain after acute injury is essential to avoid secondary brain injury. Over the last several years, multimodal monitoring has seen significant advances in the field. In this chapter, we will focus on monitoring of cerebral oxygenation and its implications on the management of critically ill brain injured patients.

The brain is a very unique organ. It has limited stores of high-energy phosphate compounds and a high metabolic demand. Hence, it is critically dependent upon a continuous flow of oxygen to meet that demand. In traumatic brain injury (TBI), intracerebral hemorrhage (ICH), and other catastrophic brain injury, it is not uncommon to observe fluctuations in oxygen delivery. Several studies have shown that brain hypoxia is associated with poor outcome (1–4). New tools currently available for advanced cerebral monitoring will allow neurointensivists to monitor brain oxygenation more accurately.

BRAIN TISSUE OXYGEN MONITORING

Techniques

There are two methods used to measure brain tissue oxygen tension ($PbtO_2$), the optical luminescent and the polarographic methods. In the optical luminescent method, oxygen molecules trigger a change in the color of Ruthenium dye. A pulse of light changes frequency as it penetrates the dye. This change in frequency is then converted into a partial pressure of oxygen. This is the method used in the Neurotrend Device (Diametrics Medical, St. Paul, Minnesota; no longer commercially available in the United States). In the polarographic method, a Clark electrode is used to measure oxygen content. Oxygen from the brain tissue diffuses across a semipermeable membrane to be reduced by a gold polarographic cathode generating a flow of electrical current proportional to the oxygen concentration. This technique was introduced for brain monitoring in 1993 (5). Using this method, the Licox Brain Oxygen Monitor (Integra Neuroscience, Plainsboro, New Jersey) was approved by the Food and Drug Administration (FDA) in the United States in 2001. Both methods measure oxygen with high accuracy with slightly higher precision in the optical luminescent method. Response times to changes in oxygen concentration tend to be slightly shorter with the optical compared to polarographic method (6,7). This slight difference does not appear to be clinically significant.

Placement

The probe is usually placed directly into the brain parenchyma with a fixed cranial bolt, approximately 2 to 3 cm below the dura, targeting frontal white matter (Figure 4.1). The tip measures the partial pressure of oxygen in a 13-mm tissue cylinder around the catheter and is, therefore, a regional monitor. Optimal probe placement location continues to be a controversial issue with variability in the generalization of data depending on whether the monitor is placed in the injured or uninjured brain (4,8). In TBI patients, most centers tend to place the monitor into normal-appearing brain tissue in the frontal lobe of the most severely injured hemisphere. When there is diffuse injury, the monitor is usually placed in the nondominant hemisphere. Some recommend placement of the tip in penumbral areas, but this remains technically difficult to identify with certainty. In subarachnoid hemorrhage (SAH) patients, the monitor is usually placed on the side of the ruptured aneurysm or the area most at risk for vasospasm. Post insertion CT confirmation of probe position is important for data interpretation. It is advisable to

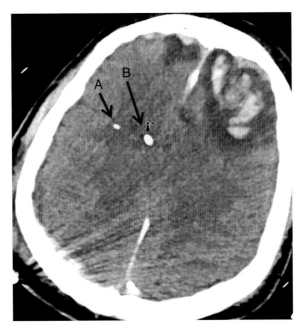

FIGURE 4.1 Axial noncontrast head CT of a patient who suffered severe TBI including frontal contusions. Arrow A marks the tip of a brain tissue oxygen probe in the right frontal lobe. Arrow B identifies a ventricular catheter.

attempt an oxygenation trial to assess changes in PbO_2 in response to increase in fraction of inspired oxygen (FiO_2). This trial helps exclude structural interference from surrounding microhemorrhages or sensor damage resulting from insertion. An equilibration of up to an hour is required in order to ensure stable readings.

Placement of the $PbtO_2$ probe carries minimal risks. Probe track hematomas are reported to occur after 1% to 2% of placements (9,10). Infectious complications are also rarely described.

INTERPRETATION AND CLINICAL UTILITY

Normal brain oxygen tension has been acquired experimentally, but human measurements have been restricted to normal values obtained during neurosurgical procedures and normal-appearing brain after TBI. Animal data revealed a range of normal $PbtO_2$ from 30 to 42 mmHg (11,12). Human recordings have varied from 37 mmHg to 48 mmHg in uncompromised patients undergoing cerebrovascular surgery (13,14). The exact $PbtO_2$ threshold that represents ischemia is not known. In the literature, ischemic thresholds have ranged between 10 and 19 mmHg (8,15,16). A threshold of 10 to 15 mmHg has been used primarily based on positron emission tomography (PET)-validated studies (17). Recently, CT perfusion mean transit time (MTT) was found to also correlate with $PbtO_2$ recordings (18).

Effect of Hypoxia on Outcome

Several studies have examined the effect of brain hypoxia on outcome in patients with SAH and TBI. In SAH patients, recurrent brain hypoxia, defined as five or more 30-minute episodes of $PbtO_2 < 10$ mmHg, was less likely to result in a good outcome (23%) compared to patients with fewer than five episodes of brain hypoxia (65%) at 3 and 6 months after SAH (3). SAH patients with infarcts were more likely to have critical hypoxic episodes than those without infarcts (19).

A systematic review of three observational studies (1,20) in TBI patients found that brain hypoxia (defined as $PbtO_2 < 10$ mmHg) was associated with increased mortality (72%) compared to patients without any evidence of hypoxia (43%). The odds ratio for death with brain hypoxia was 4 (confidence interval (CI) 1.9–8.2). Similarly, TBI patients with hypoxia had unfavorable outcome (55% vs 24%) compared to patient without hypoxia at 6 months postdischarge.

ICP-Guided Therapy Versus $PbtO_2$-Guided Therapy

Several studies compared the outcomes of patients treated with $PbtO_2$-guided therapy with those treated with standard intracranial pressure/cerebral perfusion pressure (ICP/CPP)-guided therapy. One of the earliest studies to evaluate these two goal directed approaches enrolled severe TBI patients (21). In the study, the ICP/CPP group goals were to maintain ICP less than 20 mmHg and CPP greater than 70 mmHg. In the $PbtO_2$ group, the goal was to maintain $PbtO_2$ greater than 10 mmHg by intermittently increasing CPP as needed with vasopressors and fluids. Although the outcome was better in the $PbtO_2$ group (65%) compared to the ICP/CPP group (54%), the difference did not reach statistical significance. Stiefel and colleagues published a similar retrospective review with different therapy goals (22). The CPP goal was lower (> 60 mmHg) and the $PbtO_2$ goal was higher (> 25 mmHg). In the $PbtO_2$ group, patients were treated with intermittent oxygen and blood transfusion to maintain a hemoglobin goal of greater than 10 g/dL to counteract hypoxic episodes. $PbtO_2$ goal-directed patients had a significantly lower mortality rate (25%) compared to the ICP/CPP group (34%). In 2010, the same group reported similar outcome with a $PbtO_2$ target of 20 mmHg (23). In these trials, the Licox monitors were placed into normal tissue on the more severely injured side. Although other studies had equivocal findings (24), some have demonstrated negative outcomes with $PbtO_2$ goal-directed therapy (25). In this study the goals were to maintain ICP greater than 20 mmHg and CPP greater than 60 mmHg in the ICP/CPP group. In the $PbtO_2$ group, the goal was to keep $PbtO_2$ greater than 20 mmHg. Although mortality was the same across the two groups, the $PbtO_2$ group had worse functional outcome than the ICP/CPP group.

Other Potential Clinical Applications for PbtO₂ Monitoring

Decompressive Craniectomy

A retrospective review (26) of ICP-and $PbtO_2$-monitored SAH patients who ultimately underwent surgical hemicraniectomy for intracranial hypertension, revealed a threshold decrease in $PbtO_2$ to < 10 mmHg as the first sign of deterioration. The $PbtO_2$ ischemic threshold was present an average of 13 hours prior to herniation in 45% of patients. In another study (27), patients who were hypoxic prior to hemicraniectomy were likely to have poorer outcome.

Aneurysm Surgery

Intraoperative use of $PbtO_2$ monitoring is feasible and is a sensitive indicator for cerebral ischemia in tissue at risk (28–30). $PbtO_2$ monitoring allows not only assessment of the effect of reversibility of temporary aneurysm clipping, but can also be indicative of the correct positioning of the permanent clip (28). In a study of patients undergoing craniotomy for aneurysm clipping (29), the majority of patients who required temporary clipping of the parent vessel showed reductions in $PbtO_2$, with a level of $PbtO_2$ < 8 mmHg for 30 min being predictive of cerebral infarction.

Brain Tumor

The use of $PBtO_2$ measurement in brain tumors has been investigated (31). In this study, MRI-bases stereotaxis was used to guide sensor placement into the peritumoral area prior to craniotomy. The effect of dural opening and resection on $PbtO_2$ was measured. In patients with swelling, $PbtO_2$ increased significantly with dural opening and was maintained post resection.

Arteriovenous Malformation (AVM) Surgery

Hoffman et al measured oxygenation of cerebral tissue supplied by AVM vessels in patients undergoing AVM resection (32). Low $PbtO_2$ before AVM resection suggested low perfusion and chronic hypoxia while the marked increase in $PbtO_2$ post resection indicated hyperperfusion.

THERAPEUTIC STRATEGIES

It seems clear that low $PbtO_2$ is associated with poor outcome. However, clear therapeutic strategies to address ischemic risk have not yet been fully validated. Only two prospective studies to date addressed this question. Neither found any difference between ICP/CPP and $PbtO_2$ goal-directed therapy (33,34). The ongoing BOOST II trial is exploring $PbtO_2$-directed therapy in a randomized multicenter clinical trial of severe TBI patients. Table 4.1 summarizes the different treatment strategies based on $PbtO_2$.

JUGULAR BULB OXIMETRY

Jugular bulb oximetry is a continuous global monitor that provides insight regarding cerebral oxygen utilization. The monitoring utilizes an oximeter that is placed on the tip of a flexible catheter that is introduced percutaneously in a cephalad direction within the jugular vein. The probe is often advanced through an introducer catheter that is inserted into the neck just superior to the clavicle (Figure 4.2). Venous blood within each jugular bulb arises from mixed superficial and deep drainage from both sides of the brain. Continuous oximetry provides saturation of blood that has returned from the brain. A comparison with the saturation of the arterial systemic blood allows the oxygen extraction ratio to be calculated. Normal jugular saturations (SjO2) range between 60% and 80% (35). The brain can maximally extract oxygen from around 50% of the saturated hemoglobin molecules, beyond which delivery is dependent upon perfusion to avoid dysoxia. Fiberoptic saturation measurements are commonly calibrated regularly (every 8–12 hours) by jugular venous sampling through the tip of the catheter (36). Use of the introducer sheath allows for malfunctioning catheters to be easily replaced or removed in the necessity of MRI.

Since oxygen is unable to be stored in the brain, measured SjO_2 allow inference of oxygen delivery and utilization. Low saturation values may result from low cardiac output, anemia, severe vasoconstriction, systemic hypoxia, or increased oxygen utilization. Elevated SjO_2 occur during hyperemia, significant sedation, neuronal hypometabolism and cell death, and high cardiac output. Spuriously elevated saturations may also follow caudal displacement of the catheter with contaminated drainage from the higher saturated facial venous blood. Proper jugular bulb placement should be confirmed with a lateral skull film.

SjO_2 have prognostic value after brain injury. In 116 patients suffering severe TBI desaturations were predictive of poor neurological outcome (37). Ninety percent of patients

TABLE 4.1 Therapeutic Strategies for Cerebral Hypoxia, Defined as $PbtO_2$ < 15 mmHg. Strategies Are Stratified According to Presence or Absence of Intracranial Hypertension.

ICP < 20 mmHg	ICP > 20 mmHg
■ Optimize CPP	■ Mannitol or hypertonic saline therapy
■ Enhance oxygen delivery	
▪ Transfusion	■ Hypothermia
▪ Increase FiO_2	■ Barbiturates therapy
■ Decrease core body temperature	■ Sedation and paralytics
■ Decrease hyperventilation	■ Drain CSF if indicated

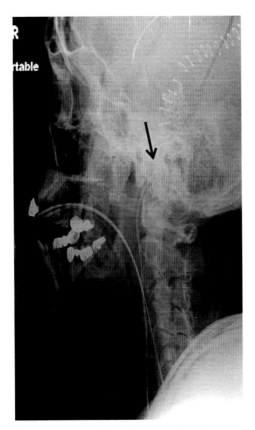

FIGURE 4.2 Lateral skull film of severe TBI patient confirming appropriate placement of a jugular bulb catheter (arrow).

with multiple prolonged (> 10 min) episodes of hypoxia were dead, severely disabled, or vegetative at 3-month follow-up, compared to a rate of 55% in patients without SjO_2 desaturations. Similarly, in a small study of aneurysmal subarachnoid hemorrhage (aSAH) patients, the oxygen extraction ratio rose 1 day prior to onset of neurological deficits related to vasospasm. Triple H therapy was successful in raising the SjO_2 in the majority of patients (38). In a study that concomitantly measured jugular bulb saturation and regional cerebral oximetry after brain injury, a distinct and complementary subset of hypoxic events were discovered with each monitor (39). Hypoxia resulting from systemic hypoxemia was detected favorably with $PbtO_2$ monitoring, whereas episodes resulting from hyperventilation were preferentially identified by SjO_2 desaturations.

There are risks and concerns related to SjO_2 monitoring. Catheter placement carries the chance of carotid artery puncture and pneumothorax due the close proximity of the lung apex to the supraclavicular jugular vein. Additionally, nonocclusive jugular vein thrombi are a recognized complication related to indwelling jugular catheters (40). Low flow rate heparinized saline perfusing through the indwelling catheter may help reduce thrombosis. While jugular oximetry is considered a global monitor, some users have reported concerns related to saturation variability during comparison of side-to-side saturation measurements (41,42). No studies have explored the clinical benefit of jugular bulb–directed therapy after brain injury. Recent literature regarding the use of jugular bulb monitoring has focused on intraoperative rather than critical care applications.

NEAR-INFRARED SPECTROSCOPY

Near-infrared spectroscopy (NIRS) is a noninvasive optical monitoring technique that utilizes infrared light to estimate brain tissue oxygenation. Infrared light is emitted from light emitting diodes and detected by silicon phosphodiode optodes placed over the scalp of the frontal lobes. The light traverses biologic tissue and its absorption at specific wavelengths correlates with the presence of biologic chromophores. The attenuation of light is concentration dependent (43). The most common biologic chromopheres are deoxyhemoglobin and oxyhemoglobin, the concentrations of which have obvious clinical relevance.

NIRS has shown promise as a monitoring device in specific medical circumstances. A variety of neurovascular procedures have demonstrated impaired regional brain oxygenation during NIRS monitoring (44). A reduction in cerebral tissue oxygen saturation ($SctO_2$) of 20% during carotid endarterectomy has been shown to have value in predicting risk of stroke (45). After cardiac arrest, patients with good 6-month functional outcomes were noted to have higher regional NIRS saturations during early resuscitation (rSO_2 68% vs 58%, $P < .01$; 46).

While NIRS technology has undergone considerable evaluation as a detection device in the operating room, the utility of NIRS within the neurocritical care unit is less developed. NIRS technique and normative saturation values vary among the different manufactured monitors. This makes comparisons difficult and standardization of monitoring protocols problematic. Furthermore, most monitors have a significant amount of overlap between normal and abnormal data. NIRS can be difficult to interpret when intracranial pathology, such as hematomas and cerebral edema, are present (47,48). Nonheme chromophores, such as melanin and bilirubin, can also confound saturation measurements. Finally, the relative ratio of venous and arterial blood within the intracranial compartment is dynamic. This poses a challenge when deciphering the meaning of saturation changes.

At present, the literature does not support a role for NIRS technology within the neurocritical care unit. Considering the important role of oxygen metabolism after acute brain injury as well as the potential benefits of minimally invasive continuous monitoring, applications for NIRS will likely continue to be sought.

REFERENCES

1. Bardt TF et al. Monitoring of brain tissue PO2 in traumatic brain injury: effect of cerebral hypoxia on outcome. *Acta Neurochir Suppl.* 1998;71:153–156.
2. Chen HI et al. Detection of cerebral compromise with multimodality monitoring in patients with subarachnoid hemorrhage. *Neurosurgery.* 2011;69(1):53–63, discussion 63.
3. Kett-White R et al. Adverse cerebral events detected after subarachnoid hemorrhage using brain oxygen and microdialysis probes. *Neurosurgery.* 2002;50(6):1213–1221, discussion 1221–1222.
4. Kiening KL et al. Brain tissue pO2-monitoring in comatose patients: implications for therapy. *Neurol Res.* 1997;19(3):233–240.
5. Maas AI et al. Monitoring cerebral oxygenation: experimental studies and preliminary clinical results of continuous monitoring of cerebrospinal fluid and brain tissue oxygen tension. *Acta Neurochir Suppl (Wien).* 1993;59:50–57.

6. Hoelper BM et al. Brain oxygen monitoring: in-vitro accuracy, long-term drift and response-time of Licox- and Neurotrend sensors. *Acta Neurochir (Wien)*, 2005;147(7):767–774, discussion 774.

7. Purins K et al. Brain tissue oxygen monitoring: a study of in vitro accuracy and stability of Neurovent-PTO and Licox sensors. *Acta Neurochir (Wien).* 2010;152(4):681–688.

8. Sarrafzadeh AS et al. Cerebral oxygenation in contusioned vs. nonlesioned brain tissue: monitoring of PtiO2 with Licox and Paratrend. *Acta Neurochir Suppl.* 1998;71:186–189.

9. Dings J, Miexensberger J, Jager A, and Klaus R. Clinical experience with 118 brain tissue oxygen partial pressure catheter probes. *Neurosurgery.* 1998;43(5):1082–1094.

10. Stewart C, Haitsma I, Zador Z, et al. The new Licox combined brain tissue oxygen and brain temperature monitor: assessment of in vitro accuracy and clinical experience in severe traumatic brain injury. *Neurosurgery.* 2008;63:1159–1165.

11. Critchley GR, Bell BA, Acute cerebral tissue oxygenation changes following experimental subarachnoid hemorrhage. *Neurol Res.* 2003;25(5):451–456.

12. Zauner A et al. Brain oxygen, CO2, pH, and temperature monitoring: evaluation in the feline brain. *Neurosurgery.* 1995;37(6):1168–1176; discussion 1176–1177.

13. Hoffman WE, Charbel FT, Edelman G. Brain tissue oxygen, carbon dioxide, and pH in neurosurgical patients at risk for ischemia. *Anesth Analg.* 1996;82(3):582586.

14. Meixensberger J et al. Studies of tissue PO2 in normal and pathological human brain cortex. *Acta Neurochir Suppl (Wien).* 1993;59:58–63.

15. Doppenberg EM, et al. Determination of the ischemic threshold for brain oxygen tension. *Acta Neurochir Suppl.* 1998;71:166–169.

16. Valadka AB et al. Relationship of brain tissue PO2 to outcome after severe head injury. *Crit Care Med.* 1998;26(9):1576–1581.

17. Johnston AJ et al. Effect of cerebral perfusion pressure augmentation with dopamine and norepinephrine on global and focal brain oxygenation after traumatic brain injury. *Intensive Care Med.* 2004;30(5):791–797.

18. Hemphill JC 3rd et al. Relationship between brain tissue oxygen tension and CT perfusion: feasibility and initial results. *AJNR Am J Neuroradiol.* 2005;26(5):1095–1100.

19. Vath A. et al., Therapeutic aspects of brain tissue pO2 monitoring after subarachnoid hemorrhage. *Acta Neurochir Suppl.* 2002;81:307–309.

20. van den Brink WA et al. Brain oxygen tension in severe head injury. *Neurosurgery.* 2000;46(4):868–876, discussion 876–878.

21. Meixensberger J et al. Brain tissue oxygen guided treatment supplementing ICP/CPP therapy after traumatic brain injury. *J Neurol Neurosurg Psychiatry.* 2003;74(6):760–764.

22. Stiefel MF et al. Reduced mortality rate in patients with severe traumatic brain injury treated with brain tissue oxygen monitoring. *J Neurosurg,* 2005:103(5):805–811.

23. Spiotta AM et al. Brain tissue oxygen-directed management and outcome in patients with severe traumatic brain injury. *J Neurosurg.* 2010;113(3):571–580.

24. Narotam PK, Morrison JF, Nathoo N. Brain tissue oxygen monitoring in traumatic brain injury and major trauma: outcome analysis of a brain tissue oxygen-directed therapy. *J Neurosurg,* 2009;111(4):672–682.

25. Martini RP et al. Management guided by brain tissue oxygen monitoring and outcome following severe traumatic brain injury. *J Neurosurg.* 2009; 111(4):644–649.

26. Strege RJ et al. Cerebral edema leading to decompressive craniectomy: an assessment of the preceding clinical and neuromonitoring trends. *Neurol Res.* 2003;25(5):510–515.

27. Stiefel MF et al. Cerebral oxygenation following decompressive hemicraniectomy for the treatment of refractory intracranial hypertension. *J Neurosurg.* 2004;101(2):241–247.

28. Gelabert-Gonzalez M, Fernandez-Villa JM, Ginesta-Galan, V. Intra-operative monitoring of brain tissue O2 (PtiO2) during aneurysm surgery. *Acta Neurochir (Wien).* 2002;144(9):863–866, discussion 866–867.

29. Kett-White R. et al. Cerebral oxygen and microdialysis monitoring during aneurysm surgery: effects of blood pressure, cerebrospinal fluid drainage, and temporary clipping on infarction. *J Neurosurg.* 2002;96(6):1013–1019.

30. Szelenyi A et al. Brain tissue oxygenation monitoring supplementary to somatosensory evoked potential monitoring for aneurysm surgery. Initial clinical experience. *Neurol Res.* 2002;24(6):555–562.

31. Pennings FA et al. Intraoperative monitoring of brain tissue oxygen and carbon dioxide pressures reveals low oxygenation in peritumoral brain edema. *J Neurosurg Anesthesiol.* 2003;15(1):1–5.

32. Hoffman WE et al. Brain tissue gases and pH during arteriovenous malformation resection. *Neurosurgery.* 1997;40(2):294–300, discussion 300–301.

33. Adamides AA et al. Focal cerebral oxygenation and neurological outcome with or without brain tissue oxygen-guided therapy in patients with traumatic brain injury. *Acta Neurochir (Wien).* 2009;151(11):1399–1409.

34. McCarthy MC et al. Neurologic outcomes with cerebral oxygen monitoring in traumatic brain injury. *Surgery.* 2009;146(4):585–590, discussion 590–591.

35. Chieregato A, Calzolari F, Trasfoini G, et al. Normal jugular bulb saturation. J *Neurol Neurosurg Psychiatry.* 2003;74(6):784–786.

36. Coplin WM, O'Keefe GE, Grady MS, et al. Accuracy of continuous jugular bulb oximetry in the intensive care unit. *Neurosurgery.* 1998;42(3):533–540.

37. Gopinath SP, Robertson CS, Contant CF, et al. Jugular venous desaturation and outcome after head injury. *J Neurol Neurosurg Psychiatry.* 1994;57:717–723.

38. Heran NS, Hentschel SJ, and Toyota BD Jugular Bulb Oximetry for Prediction of Vasospasm Following Subarachnoid Hemorrhage. *Can J Neurol Sci.* 2004;31:80–86.

39. Gopinath SP, Valadka AB, Masahiko U, et al. Comparison of jugular venous oxygen saturation and brain tissue PO_2 as monitors of cerebral ischemia after head injury. *Crit Care Med.* 1999;27(11):2337–2345.

40. Coplin WM, O'Keefe GE, Grady MS, et al. Thrombotic, infectious, and procedural complications of the jugular bulb catheter in the intensive care unit. *Neurosurgery.* 1997;41(1):101–109.

41. Metz C, Holzschuh M, Bein T, et al. Monitoring of cerebral oxygen metabolism in the jugular bulb: reliability of unilateral measurements in severe head injury. *J Cereb Blood Flow Metab.* 1998;18:332–343.

42. Nicola L, Beindorf AE, Rasulo F, et al. Limits of intermittent jugular bulb oxygen saturation monitoring in the management of severe head trauma patients. *Neurosurgery.* 2000;46(5):1131–1139.

43. Ghosh A, Elwell C, Smith M. Cerebral near-infrared spectroscopy in adults: a work in progress. *Anesth Anlg.* 2012;115:1373–1383.

44. Nielsen HB. Systematic review of near-infrared spectroscopy determined cerebral oxygenation during non-cardiac surgery. *Frontiers in Physiology.* 2014;5(93):1–15.

45. Mille T, Tachimiri ME, Klersy C, et al. Near infrared spectroscopy monitoring during carotid endarterectomy: which threshold value is critical? *Eur J Vasc Endovasc Surg.* 2004;27:646–650.

46. Storm C, Leithner C, Krannich A, et al. Regional cerebral oxygen saturation after cardiac arrest in 60 patients—A prospective outcome study. Resuscitation. 2014 Apr 30. Pii:S0300-9572(14)00507-3. Doi:10.1016/j [Epub ahead of print].

47. Robertson CS, Gopinath SP, and Chance B. A new application for near-infrared spectroscopy: detection of delayed intracranial hematomas after head injury. *J Neurotrauma.* 1995;12:591–600.

48. Gill AS, Rajneesh KF, Owen CM, et al. Early optical detection of cerebral edema in vivo. *J Neurosurg.* 2011;114:470–477.

Brain Tissue Perfusion Monitoring

David M. Panczykowski, MD
Lori Shutter, MD

INTRODUCTION

The ultimate determinant of oxygenation and substrate delivery to the brain is cerebral perfusion. Although mean arterial pressure (MAP) is the primary driving force for tissue perfusion, cerebral blood flow (CBF) is determined by multiple intrinsic factors. Systemic perfusion monitoring in the critically ill population (eg, invasive arterial blood pressure, oxygen saturation of blood, etc) is vital for detecting global changes; however, management of patients with cerebral pathology specifically requires accurate understanding of CBF. Since the purpose of many interventions in the neurologic ICU is based on augmenting arterial blood flow, information provided by brain-specific perfusion monitoring can be extremely helpful in guiding clinical management. The assessment and regulation of an individual patient's CBF has been made possible by the introduction of several techniques to measure brain perfusion.

Types of Monitors Available for Brain Tissue Perfusion Assessment

Techniques to assess cerebral perfusion have existed for decades, but it is only recently that continuous, bedside monitoring has been available. Measurement of cerebral perfusion can be divided numerous ways, including quantitative versus qualitative assessment, dynamic versus static, invasive versus noninvasive (see Table 5.1). Although a myriad of monitoring options exist, the optimal method has yet to be determined. Zauner and coworkers summarized the criteria of the ideal method for monitoring brain-injured patients as follows: It should be continuous, quantitative, applicable to bedside use, sensitive enough to detect harmful events, non- or minimally invasive, robust, user-friendly, and cost effective (1).

TABLE 5.1 Summary of the More Common Modalities for Brain Tissue Perfusion Monitoring

MODALITY	PROS	CONS
Imaging		
Xenon-CT	High spatial resolution	Requires special equipment and technicians
		Requires transport
CT Perfusion	High spatial resolution	Influenced by regional vessel density and diameter
	Available anywhere with CT scanner	Cannot be used in patients with iodinated contrast allergy
	Lower radiation dose than Xe-CT	Requires transport
	Shorter time interval between successive scans	Cannot be used in patients with renal insufficiency
Invasive monitoring		
Thermal Diffusion Probe	High temporal resolution	Invasive
	Can be integrated with other modalities of neuromonitoring	Only measures tissue within a volume of ~27 mm³
	Can be used at the bedside	Cannot be used in febrile (> 39.5°C) patients
	Immediate, goal-directed treatment feedback	

Currently available imaging modalities for the measurement of cerebral perfusion include xenon-enhanced computed tomography (Xe-CT), computed tomography perfusion (CTP), single photon emission computed tomography (SPECT), positron emission tomography (PET), and MRI perfusion. The accepted gold standard for CBF measurement has been stable Xe-CT, which has been used for more than 20 years to quantitatively evaluate CBF in humans. This technique is based on equations established during early human CBF studies by Kety and Schmidt in the 1940s. The Kety–Schmidt principle assumes that the rate of uptake and clearance of an inert diffusible tracer is proportional to blood flow in that tissue. To perform this imaging study, patients are ventilated using a xenon–oxygen mixture and successive scans are obtained to derive a curve of enhancement over time. A CBF map is then calculated from the arterial and tissue xenon time curves, using the Kety–Schmidt equation (2). Based on similar principles, CTP with iodinated contrast has increasingly supplanted Xe-CT to yield quantitative information about CBF, mean transit-time (MTT) or time to peak (TTP), and cerebral blood volume (CBV). This technique involves sequential scans through selected regions during IV administration of iodinated contrast material. Major advantages over Xe-CT are that CTP can be easily performed at any institution with a CT unit, does not require specialized material or technicians, and can be performed quickly in acutely affected patients. Obvious drawbacks of both Xe-CT and CTP, as well as other neuroimaging techniques, are that they cannot be routinely performed at bedside and only provide a time- and region-specific snapshot of CBF. Furthermore, imaging techniques require critically ill patients leave the ICU, thus introducing the inherent risks of transport.

Transcranial Doppler (TCD) ultrasonography, which measures mean blood flow velocity in the major cerebral vessels, is routinely employed as an indirect assessment of cerebral perfusion at the bedside. The Doppler shift principle is employed to derive red blood cell flow velocities from measurements of pulsed US waves insonated through various bone "windows" (eg, transtemporal through the thin, temporal squamosa above the zygomatic arch). Changes in CBF are inferred from changes in blood flow velocity (assuming a constant vessel diameter and angle of insonation; 3,4). Although TCD ultrasonography can provide noninvasive, real-time data, only flow velocities in the major cerebral arteries can be measured; thus, tissue perfusion abnormalities at the microcirculatory level may be missed. Other drawbacks include dependence on operator expertise and difficulty with cumbersome probe fixation for continuous monitoring. For these reasons, the practicality of TCD monitoring of CBF remains limited (5).

Laser Doppler (LD) flowmetry utilizes measurement principles similar to those of TCD ultrasonography; however, LD flowmetry permits assessment of microcirculatory changes. A 0.5 to 1 mm diameter fiberoptic laser probe placed on the cortical surface or in white matter emits and detects a monochromatic laser light reflected by moving red blood cells to derive flow velocity. This provides continuous, qualitative estimates of regional CBF displayed in arbitrary perfusion units. Changes in LD flowmetry correlate with alterations in cerebral perfusion pressure (CPP) and can predict impairments of autoregulation (6). Major disadvantages to LD flowmetry are that information on CBF is provided only in relative terms and data output is prone to artifacts produced by movement or probe migration (7).

Thermal diffusion (TD) flowmetry is the only modality that provides continuous, quantitative brain tissue perfusion measurement. This technique uses an intraparenchymal microprobe that measures a tissue's heat conduction and convection properties to quantitatively estimate regional tissue perfusion in absolute CBF values (0–200 mL/100 g/min). A probe containing two thermistors is inserted into brain parenchyma and measures the tissue's ability to dissipate heat, and the dissipation of heat is proportional to blood flow in the tissue over approximately a 27 mm^3 region surrounding the probe tip. TD flowmetry provides continuous, bedside CBF measurement and has been shown to be comparable to Xe-CT scanning in both animal and human studies (8). However, like all regional monitors, TD flowmetry may not accurately reflect global CBF or even local perfusion in areas with dissimilar vasoreactivity or baseline CBF.

Literature Supporting Cerebral Perfusion Monitoring

Altered brain tissue perfusion is common throughout the spectrum of illness encountered in the neurologic ICU and leads to ischemic injury and/or hyperemia with ensuing edema.

These alterations may be secondary to extrinsic perfusion problems (systemic hypotension) and/or intrinsic factors (impaired autoregulation or vasospasm). Although the importance of providing adequate blood flow to the injured brain is obvious, no randomized trial has yet evaluated whether direct monitoring leads to improved outcomes.

CPP has been used as an index of the input pressure determining CBF with several studies in the literature on traumatic brain injury (TBI) evaluating perfusion-targeted management strategies. Results have been mixed, although they seem to demonstrate a dependence on autoregulation status. Perfusion-targeted approaches have shown superior outcomes in patients with intact autoregulation, while the contrary has been true in those with impaired autoregulation, where intracranial pressure (ICP)-directed management has conferred better outcomes (9). In addition, indiscriminate maintenance of CPP greater than 70 mmHg has been associated with increased ICP, acute respiratory distress syndrome (ARDS), and mortality. Thus, the most recent *Guidelines for the Management of Severe TBI* (25) recommend CPP values within a range of 50 to 70 mmHg, with those patients demonstrating intact autoregulation often tolerating higher CPP values (10). These results suggest that at a minimum, cerebral perfusion treatment strategies should be based on an individual's cerebrovascular characteristics, and specifically autoregulation status may be an important factor in determining how best to optimize CBF. However, CPP merely reflects a general pressure gradient that is not a substitute for quantifying CBF. In both these and recent American Heart Association and Neurocritical Care *SAH Guidelines* (26), no mention is made of the optimal method of CBF or autoregulatory monitoring (11).

Studies in subarachnoid hemorrhage (SAH), ischemic stroke, and TBI have demonstrated utility of neuroimaging methods for direct assessment of CBF utilizing xenon imaging, SPECT, PET scanning, and perfusion MRI. Xe-CT has allowed evaluation of the heterogeneity of flow alterations after TBI, manipulation of PCO_2 in patients with intracranial hypertension, and blood pressure elevation for the treatment of cerebral vasospasm. More recently, quantitative CBF measurement by CTP has been shown to be consistent within individuals and has been validated by comparison with other techniques such as microspheres, Xe-CT, and PET (12). Extensive literature in the setting of acute stroke has provided clinical validation of CTP by comparison with other imaging techniques to predict areas of ischemic but salvageable and infarcted brain (12,13). CT perfusion has been shown to be 95% accurate in demonstrating the extent of supratentorial infarcts (4). These techniques have been subsequently translated into CBF surveillance and treatment of ischemia caused by vasospasm. In a recent meta-analysis for prediction of angiographic vasospasm, the sensitivity of CTP was 74%, with 93% sensitivity. While these techniques may represent the current gold standard for measurement of CBF, they cannot provide continuous monitoring.

Brain tissue perfusion measurements utilizing TD flowmetry have been applied to patients following SAH and TBI, as well as intraoperatively during tumor resection, aneurysm clipping, and arteriovenous malformation (AVM) resection. Carter and Atkinson were the first to report use of an on-lay cortical sensor for measurement of CBF in quantitative values (14). Despite reports of reliable regional cortical blood flow measurements, this technique was not generally accepted due to technical and methodological difficulties. In 2000, Vajkoczy et al reported on the validity of a novel TD flowmetry probe inserted into brain parenchyma, similar to current ICP and partial brain tissue oxygen ($PbtO_2$) monitors (Thermal Diffusion Probe, Hemedex; Cambridge, Massachusetts). Since these initial studies, several other investigations have demonstrated good agreement between TD flowmetry and Xe-CT for regional CBF measurement (8). In patients suffering SAH, TD flowmetry has been shown to reliably detect development of cerebral vasospasm-associated hypoperfusion (8,10,15). Jaeger et al demonstrated a strong correlation between TD flowmetry assessment of CBF and brain tissue oxygenation following both high-grade SAH and severe TBI (16). They found that the level of $PbtO_2$ seems to be predominately determined by regional CBF, since changes in $PbtO_2$ correlated with CBF in 90% of episodes. TD probes have also been used in multimodal neuromonitoring after TBI to evaluate individual hemodynamic parameters, including vasoreactivity, thus allowing guidance of optimal MAP and CPP therapy (17,18).

Pathophysiology

The ultimate goal of neuromonitoring is to provide an optimal environment to reduce or prevent secondary injury and promote recovery. Brain ischemia and hypoxia are central causes of damage following cerebral injury. Injured neuronal cells demonstrate increased metabolic activation, while cerebral perfusion is often impaired over the same period of time, leading to an imbalance in supply and demand. Normal global CBF is approximately 50 mL/100 g/min (approximately 80 mL/100 g/min in gray matter and 20 mL/100 g/min in white matter). Protein synthesis in neurons ceases when the CBF falls below 35 mL/100 g/min, electrical or synaptic failure occurs and neurons shift to anaerobic metabolism at or below 20 mL/100 g/min, and metabolic failure and cell death occur at or below 10 mL/100 g/min. The ultimate degree of ischemic cerebral damage depends on the magnitude of reduced blood flow, duration of insult, region specific vulnerability, and a wide variety of other factors (glycemic stores, temperature, etc). The relationship of CBF to blood pressure and vascular resistance is demonstrated by the equation CBF = CPP/CVR, where CPP (the difference between MAP and ICP) is divided by cerebrovascular resistance (CVR). During normal physiologic conditions, both flow-metabolism coupling and myogenic mechanisms finely regulate CVR, ensuring that CBF is adequate to meet cerebral oxidative metabolic demands despite fluctuations in systemic perfusion pressure. However, when cerebral autoregulation is impaired, as is often the case after brain injury, CBF is dependent upon CPP, thus predisposing the patient to cerebral ischemia and/or hyperemia.

CLINICAL ASPECTS OF MONITORING BRAIN TISSUE PERFUSION

Which Patients Would Benefit From Monitoring?

Monitoring in the neurologic ICU can be divided into general (systemic) and brain-specific methods. Although systemic monitoring is crucial for surveillance of global pathophysiology, brain-specific monitoring techniques enable more focused assessment of secondary insults that may otherwise go undetected, especially in comatose and/or pharmacologically sedated patients. While a number of pathologic situations may benefit from additional monitoring, specific scenarios carry a greater chance of disturbed cerebral perfusion and autoregulation, thus outweighing any associated risk of monitoring. The most common disease processes that may produce disturbed cerebral perfusion include ischemic stroke, TBI, and aneurysmal SAH. Cerebral perfusion may also be worsened by any pathology leading to intracranial hypertension (eg, postoperative cerebral edema, intraparenchymal hemorrhage, etc.).

A primary objective of monitoring brain tissue perfusion is identification of tissue at risk for infarction that may benefit from restoration of blood flow through direct or indirect intervention before irreversible damage occurs. In addition, monitoring may assist in differentiating cortical ischemia from hyperemia, and permit autoregulation and CO_2 reactivity tests to be done permitting tailored cerebral perfusion strategies. The following are general recommendations regarding the timing and conditions under which monitoring should be considered:

1. SAH or TBI with a Glasgow Coma Score (GCS) < 9 following adequate pulmonary and hemodynamic resuscitation

2. SAH or TBI with a GCS < 9 in whom other intracranial monitors (ICP, $PbtO_2$, etc) will be placed

3. SAH or TBI with a persistent GCS < 9 during the initial 5 to 10 days following injury (not explained by cerebral edema, hydrocephalus, seizure, fever, infection, etc)

4. SAH or TBI with neurologic deterioration, ICP elevation, $PbtO_2$ decline, or worsening of EEG and/or other monitor of brain function within the initial 14 days of injury

Phasic alterations in CBF may occur immediately following and for up to 14 days after TBI, stemming from systemic hypoperfusion, hyperemia, and vasospasm. Studies evaluating severe TBI have demonstrated that ischemia may occur in the acute post injury phase in as many as 35% of patients independent of systemic hypotension (19). Complicating this fact is that cerebral autoregulation may also be impaired, making CBF assessment very useful for early monitoring and treatment guidance. Both Xe-CT and CTP have been utilized to characterize heterogeneity of CBF alterations after TBI, providing insight into therapies designed to improve CBF as well as guide management of ICP and CPP. Monitoring of CBF beyond 12 to 24 hours remains necessary for identification of hyperemia due to impaired autoregulation and early detection of ischemia secondary to cerebral vasospasm. Rosenthal et al utilized TD flowmetry to demonstrate impaired CBF reactivity to MAP challenge in 53% of severe TBI patients (17). Following a time course similar to SAH, cerebral vasospasm may develop in up to 40% of severe TBI patients, occurring most frequently between days 4 and 14 (20).

Similar to TBI, aneurysmal SAH is associated with temporal fluctuations in cerebral perfusion. Acute alterations in CBF may be a consequence of acute vasospasm, thrombosis of the aneurysm with extension into the parent vessel or downstream embolism, or a transient reduction in CPP related to increased ICP at the time of bleeding. Although vasospasm is the most common etiology of CBF aberrancy following SAH, impaired cerebrovascular autoregulation may also predispose this population to hyperemic insult. Angiographic vasospasm of proximal intracranial vessels occurs in up to 70% of SAH patients, while 20% to 40% will experience delayed ischemic neurologic deterioration, many without an angiographic correlate. Routine brain perfusion monitoring is of greatest utility in those with limited neurologic exams where clinical parameters and crude scales lack the sensitivity to detect secondary ischemic insults and up to 20% of patients may go on to suffer unrecognized infarcts (21).

Placement of Thermal Diffusion Monitors

The TD flowmetry probe is typically placed in the least-injured hemisphere in tissue most at risk for secondary ischemic injury. Care should be taken to ensure that the probe is not placed within a contusion, infarct, or hematoma, as the goal is to prevent secondary injury to tissue at risk, and not assess tissue that has already suffered irreversible damage. For implantation, a one-way bolt is inserted through a 3.2 mm burr hole placed at or just anterior to the coronal suture and 2 to 3 cm lateral to midline (roughly at Kocher's point; Figure 5.1). This location allows assessment of the watershed zone between the anterior and middle cerebral arteries, and avoids the eloquent cortex (the motor strip is 4 to 5 cm posterior to the coronal suture). The probe is inserted subcortically to a depth of 2 to 2.5 cm below the dura mater and secured by tightening the bolt. In this location the probe can be placed employing the same incision used for the ventriculostomy drain or intraparenchymal monitor placement. Different locations may be more suitable depending on the vascular region of interest, particularly in patients suffering SAH where the arterial territories most likely to experience vasospasm and delayed cerebral ischemia are those perfused by the ruptured artery. A post procedure CT scan should be taken to ensure proper placement

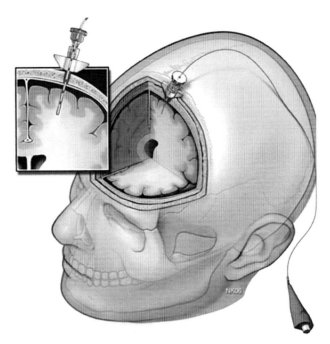

FIGURE 5.1 Illustration of frontal placement of QFlow 500™ (Hemedex, Cambridge, Massachusetts) Thermal Diffusion Probe fixed with a cranial bolt. Courtesy of Frank Bowman, PhD. Hemedex, Inc. Cambridge, Massachusetts.

of the probe. Several studies have performed CT perfusion immediately following monitor placement to record concordance between modalities; however, this is not required.

There have been no multicenter trials evaluating the complication risk of invasive neuromonitoring, or specifically CBF monitoring. Reported complications of similar intraparenchymal monitors include intracerebral, subdural, or epidural hemorrhage, meningitis, malfunction, or misplacement. These risks are less than 2%, with even fewer clinically significant complications (22).

What Are the Conventionally Accepted Monitoring Thresholds That Should Prompt Clinical Intervention?

At this time, optimal brain tissue perfusion thresholds for the initiation, titration, and withdrawal of treatment are unknown due to a lack of prospective trials investigating treatment modification on outcome. CBF in white matter is expected to range between 18 and 25 mL/100 g/min, compared with the mean global CBF ranging between 40 and 50 mL/100 g/min. Flow at or below 10 mL/100g/min typically leads to loss of neuronal integrity and infarction.

Stable Xe-CT and CTP have been routinely used to distinguish tissue at risk for infarction following ischemic stroke, and these techniques have been subsequently translated into surveillance and treatment of ischemia caused by vasospasm following TBI and SAH. Side-to-side differences in perfusion or absolute thresholds of CBF and MTT can be used to distinguish the presence of treatable, ischemic brain from infarct. Data from the stroke literature have set thresholds for salvageable tissue ranging from CBF less than 30% to 50% of an analogous region in the contralateral hemisphere defined as healthy on the basis of clinical symptomatology. Another method is to evaluate MTT and CBV maps. In regions of prolonged MTT, increases in CBV (from vasodilation and recruitment) occur where autoregulation is preserved, while decreased CBV corresponds to areas having already undergone infarction.

Regional CBF monitoring allows real-time detection of ischemia secondary to vasospasm, even before clinical signs develop. Thresholds for diagnosis of symptomatic vasospasm have been applied to TD flowmetry monitoring. Vajkoczy et al employed a cutoff value of 15 mL/100 g/min for vasospasm diagnosis and found that none of the patients with symptomatic vasospasm were missed by TD flowmetry (sensitivity 100%, specificity 75%). In addition, alterations in TD flowmetry preceded clinical evidence of vasospasm by an average of 3 days (15) (see Figure 5.2).

In management of aneurysmal SAH, hypertension with normovolemia is a mainstay of cerebral vasospasm treatment with CBF being a primary endpoint in both research and clinical settings (21). Using Xe-CT to measure CBF, Darby et al demonstrated dopamine-induced hypertension increased CBF in ischemic, noninfarcted territories without producing an increase in mean global CBF (23). On the other hand, prophylactic hypervolemic therapy has demonstrated no difference between mean global CBF, minimal regional CBF, or symptomatic spasm. Given the attendant risks, including the possibility of cardiac failure, electrolyte abnormality, cerebral edema, and bleeding diathesis resulting from dilution of clotting factors, the American Heart Association and Neurocritical Care *SAH*

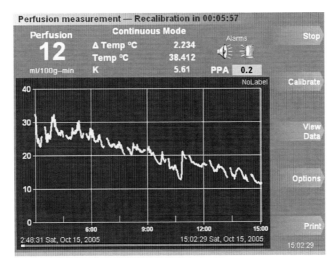

FIGURE 5.2 Screen display from Bowman Perfusion Monitor with downward trending CBF (mL/100 g-min) and the patient's associated CT-perfusion demonstrating CBF deficit in the right frontal lobe (mL/100 g-min). Angiography confirmed cerebral vasospasm secondary to aneurysmal SAH. Courtesy of Stephen Lewis, MD, University of Florida.

Guidelines have determined that prophylactic hyperdynamic therapy should be avoided (11,21). Although no discrete threshold exists, it appears relatively certain that induced arterial hypertension may be extremely useful in reversing CBF deficits once they occur. In a study utilizing TD flowmetry, Muench et al demonstrated vasopressor-induced elevation of MAP caused a significant increase of regional CBF and brain tissue oxygenation in all patients with SAH (10). In addition to the quantitative assessment of CBF, TD flowmetry allows assessment of cerebrovascular resistance providing information on vasospasm severity by considering the CPP necessary to achieve certain perfusion parameters.

Cerebral autoregulation and CO_2 reactivity may also be assessed in patients with severe TBI using TD flowmetry by calculating the response to MAP and hyperventilation challenges. Increases or decreases in cerebrovascular resistance with MAP challenges may be a simple provocative test to determine patients' autoregulatory status following severe TBI. TD flowmetry may thus improve CBF management after TBI by optimizing MAP, CPP, and ICP targets through assessment of cerebral autoregulation (24).

Although modality specific thresholds exist for the diagnosis of impaired CBF and may be associated with outcome, all available data, including trends, should be integrated before making treatment decisions.

SUMMARY

The optimal treatment of neurologic injury requires the prevention and amelioration of secondary insults, with none more important than altered cerebral perfusion. Qualitative modalities such as TCD or LD flowmetry permit bedside trending of CBF surrogates. Quantitative assessment produces easily understood implementable data that can be obtained through either imaging with Xe-CT and CTP, or at the bedside with regional TD flowmetry. Monitoring brain tissue perfusion permits early detection of ischemia and assessment of autoregulation. This allows prompt diagnosis and management of secondary insults and the individualization of treatment protocols through optimizing systemic blood pressure goals. Furthermore, continuous CBF monitoring provides real-time analysis of treatment effects and the interactions comorbid conditions and interventions have on cerebral perfusion. Substantial evidence supports the diagnostic accuracy of these CBF monitoring modalities; however, few studies have evaluated their ideal implementation and potential impact on outcome. Regardless, the importance of adequate cerebral perfusion is implicit, as is the necessity of its vigilant monitoring in the neurologic ICU.

REFERENCES

1. Zauner A, Bullock R, Di X, et al. Brain oxygen, CO2, pH, and temperature monitoring: evaluation in the feline brain. *Neurosurgery*. 1995;37(6):1168–1176; discussion 76–77.
2. Yonas H, Darby JM, Marks EC, et al. CBF measured by Xe-CT: approach to analysis and normal values. *J Cereb Blood Flow Metab*. 1991;11(5):716–725.
3. Dahl A, Russell D, Nyberg-Hansen R, et al. A comparison of regional cerebral blood flow and middle cerebral artery blood flow velocities: simultaneous measurements in healthy subjects. *J Cereb Blood Flow Metab*. 1992;12(6):1049–1054.
4. Wintermark M, Sesay M, Barbier E, et al. Comparative overview of brain perfusion imaging techniques. *J Neuroradiol*. 2005;32(5):294–314.
5. Bhatia A, Gupta AK. Neuromonitoring in the intensive care unit. I. Intracranial pressure and cerebral blood flow monitoring. *Intensive Care Med*. 2007;33(7):1263–1271.
6. Arbit E, DiResta GR. Application of laser Doppler flowmetry in neurosurgery. *Neurosurg Clin N Am*. 1996;7(4):741–748.
7. Obeid AN, Barnett NJ, Dougherty G, et al. A critical review of laser Doppler flowmetry. *J Med Eng Technol*. 1990;14(5):178–181.
8. Vajkoczy P, Roth H, Horn P, et al. Continuous monitoring of regional cerebral blood flow: experimental and clinical validation of a novel thermal diffusion microprobe. *J Neurosurg*. 2000;93(2): 265–274.
9. Howells T, Elf K, Jones PA, et al. Pressure reactivity as a guide in the treatment of cerebral perfusion pressure in patients with brain trauma. *J Neurosurg*. 2005;102(2):311–317.
10. Muench E, Horn P, Bauhuf C, et al. Effects of hypervolemia and hypertension on regional cerebral blood flow, intracranial pressure, and brain tissue oxygenation after subarachnoid hemorrhage. *Crit Care Med*. 2007;35(8):1844–1851; quiz 52.
11. Bederson JB, Connolly ES, Jr., Batjer HH, et al. Guidelines for the management of aneurysmal subarachnoid hemorrhage: a statement for healthcare professionals from a special writing group of the Stroke Council, American Heart Association. *Stroke*. 2009;40(3):994–1025.
12. Harrigan MR, Leonardo J, Gibbons KJ, et al. CT perfusion cerebral blood flow imaging in neurological critical care. *Neurocrit Care*. 2005;2(3):352–366.
13. Wintermark M, Reichhart M, Thiran JP, et al. Prognostic accuracy of cerebral blood flow measurement by perfusion computed tomography, at the time of emergency room admission, in acute stroke patients. *Ann Neurol*. 2002;51(4):417–432.
14. Carter LP, Atkinson JR. Cortical blood flow in controlled hypotension as measured by thermal diffusion. *J Neurol Neurosurg Psychiatry*. 1973;36(6):906–913. PMCID: 1083589.
15. Vajkoczy P, Horn P, Thome C, et al. Regional cerebral blood flow monitoring in the diagnosis of delayed ischemia following aneurysmal subarachnoid hemorrhage. *J Neurosurg*. 2003;98(6): 1227–1234.
16. Jaeger M, Soehle M, Schuhmann MU, et al. Correlation of continuously monitored regional cerebral blood flow and brain tissue oxygen. *Acta Neurochir* (Wien). 2005;147(1):51–56; discussion 6.
17. Rosenthal G, Sanchez-Mejia RO, Phan N, et al. Incorporating a parenchymal thermal diffusion cerebral blood flow probe in bedside assessment of cerebral autoregulation and vasoreactivity in patients with severe traumatic brain injury. *J Neurosurg*. 2011;114(1):62–70.

18. Soukup J, Bramsiepe I, Brucke M, et al. Evaluation of a bedside monitor of regional CBF as a measure of CO2 reactivity in neurosurgical intensive care patients. *J Neurosurg Anesthesiol.* 2008;20(4):249–255.

19. Eker C, Asgeirsson B, Grande PO, et al. Improved outcome after severe head injury with a new therapy based on principles for brain volume regulation and preserved microcirculation. *Crit Care Med.* 1998;26(11):1881–1886.

20. Lee JH, Martin NA, Alsina G, et al. Hemodynamically significant cerebral vasospasm and outcome after head injury: a prospective study. *J Neurosurg.* 1997;87(2):221–233.

21. Diringer MN, Bleck TP, Claude Hemphill J, III, et al. Critical care management of patients following aneurysmal subarachnoid hemorrhage: recommendations from the Neurocritical Care Society's Multidisciplinary Consensus Conference. *Neurocrit Care.* 2011;15(2):211–240.

22. Morton R, Lucas TH, II, Ko A, et al. Intracerebral abscess associated with the Camino intracranial pressure monitor: case report and review of the literature. *Neurosurgery.* 2012;71(1):E193–E198.

23. Darby JM, Yonas H, Marks EC, et al. Acute cerebral blood flow response to dopamine-induced hypertension after subarachnoid hemorrhage. *J Neurosurg.* 1994;80(5):857–864.

24. Oddo M, Villa F, Citerio G. Brain multimodality monitoring: an update. *Curr Opin Crit Care.* 2012;18(2):111–118.

25. Guidelines for the management of severe traumatic brain injury. *J Neurotrauma* 2007;24(Suppl 1):S1-S106.

26. Connolly ES, Rabinstein AA, Carhuapoma JR, et al. Guidelines for the Management of Aneurysmal Subarachnoid Hemorrhage: a guideline for Healthcare Professionals From the American Heart Association / American Stroke Association. *Stroke.* 2012;43(6):1711–37.

Cerebral Microdialysis

Chad M. Miller, MD

INTRODUCTION

Cerebral microdialysis is a brain monitoring technique that allows real-time quantification of an array of analyte concentrations from the interstitial space of the brain. It is one of the more versatile and informative monitors available to intensivists who care for brain-injured patients. Despite its use for the past 20 years, potential applications and insights into the device's neurochemical findings are still being discovered and formulated.

FUNCTION AND DESIGN

Cerebral microdialysis is performed by placing a thin (0.9 mm) catheter with a semipermeable membrane into the white matter of the brain parenchyma. The catheter may be placed as part of a single or multilumen bolt system or independently placed through a tunneled technique. The catheter has input and output tubing leading to the membrane. A low protein solution with osmolar and electrolyte properties similar to cerebral spinal fluid (CSF) is infused into the input tubing by a battery-operated pump. The fluid passes through the membranous portion of the catheter and is collected in an exchangeable and disposable microvial, which connects to the output tubing. The perfusate solution does not extravasate into the brain interstitium or alter its volume. Rather, the constituents of the interstitium pass through the semipermeable membrane down their concentration gradients and are collected in the microdialysis tubing in a process that is driven by passive diffusion. The microvial, with its collected fluid, is then removed and placed into a portable analyzer within the critical care unit that determines the concentrations of the desired analytes (Figure 6.1). Fluid is commonly analyzed on an hourly basis. Analyte concentrations collected within the first 2 hours after catheter placement may demonstrate abnormalities related to transient tissue injury and should generally not be used in clinical decision making. The most commonly assayed analytes are glucose, pyruvate,

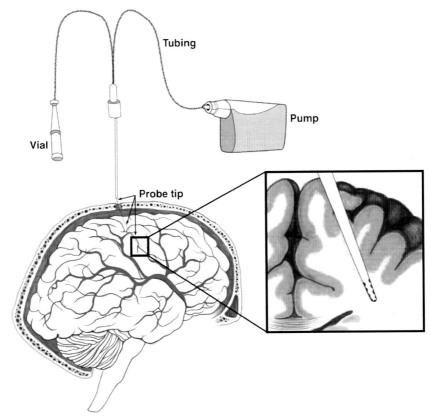

FIGURE 6.1 Schematic demonstrating a typical microdialysis neuromonitoring system. A battery-operated pump perfuses fluid though the input tubing to the microdialysis membrane on the distal tip of the implanted probe. Interstitial brain analytes diffuse down their concentration gradients through the pores in the membrane and are returned by the tubing to the collection microvial. The solution can then be quantified by a microdialysis analyzer.

lactate, glycerol, and glutamate. For these basic analytes, their collected concentration is approximately 70% of the actual concentration in the interstitial fluid (1). The efficiency of recovery depends upon the perfusion rate, membrane length, membrane pore size, and dimensions and charge of the collected analyte. Standard microdialysis techniques utilize a 10-mm long membrane with a 20 kDa pore size (M dialysis North Chelmsford, Massachusetts) perfused at a rate of 0.3 μL/min. This approach can be varied to allow better assessment of atypical analytes. A 100-kDa catheter is available for collection of larger molecules.

In recent years there has been increased interest in expanding the use of cerebral microdialysis to assay endogenous cytokines, central nervous system (CNS) penetration of medications, and a variety of other nontraditional macromolecules. Efficiency of recovery must be determined for these techniques to yield quantifiable data. Multiple different approaches have been used to discover the absolute concentration of new analytes. Variation in the perfusate rate during sample collection allows extrapolation with a fitted line to determine concentrations at zero flow rate (2). The zero flow rate is then assumed to approximate true interstitial concentration. The "no net flux" method involves inclusion of the analyte of interest in the perfusing solution with observed variation of the concentration until no net flux is seen down the concentration gradient (2). Alternatively, recovery can be determined by an in-vitro approach. Retrodialysis determines absolute concentration by testing recovery in known concentrations of analyte solution. For cytokines, this method often requires use of a colloid perfusate to limit unintended shifts of perfusate volume out of the catheter. Use of a colloid perfusate in vivo has the potential to result in regional extracellular dehydration (3).

Examination of the standard analytes (glucose, lactate, pyruvate, glutamate, and glycerol) provide important information regarding neuronal integrity, cerebral metabolic distress, and the general metabolic state of the injured brain. Given the rate and ease of transportation across the blood–brain barrier, glucose is the preferred fuel source of the brain. After the conversion of glucose to pyruvate through glycolysis, the neuronal environment determines the course and efficiency of further metabolism. In aerobic conditions, the mitochondria convert pyruvate to acetyl-CoA, which enters the citric acid cycle and produces 36 ATP through oxidation. In anaerobic conditions, pyruvate is converted to lactate to allow additional glycolysis, but without the benefit of energy production comparable to aerobic metabolism. Intracellular lactate levels increase with respect to pyruvate, both of which freely diffuse out of the cell. Consequently, elevated lactate pyruvate ratios (LPR) collected through cerebral microdialysis can be representative of anaerobic metabolism. This is particularly true in the setting of low brain glucose levels. A LPR greater than 25 is viewed as abnormal, and a value greater than 40 may represent a concerning degree of ischemia (1). An elevated LPR in the setting of ischemia or hypoxia is termed a Type I LPR. LPR elevations can also denote metabolic distress that is not ischemic in origin. This Type II LPR elevation has been described after traumatic brain injury (TBI) and aneurysmal subarachnoid hemorrhage (aSAH). Type II LPR results from reduced pyruvate that may occur related to dysfunction of the glycolytic pathway. Other described causes of Type II LPR include congenital and acquired mitochondrial dysfunction, sepsis, citric acid cycle enzymatic abnormalities, hyperammonemia, seizures, increased glycogenolysis from medication-induced metabolism, and halothane and other anesthetic/hypnotic use. Recently, there has been heightened interest in metabolic states following brain injury during which hypoglycemia may stimulate elevation in lactate related to its transport as an alternative energy source (1).

Glutamate is a recognized marker of metabolic distress, the concentrations of which are crucial in mechanisms related to brain edema, calcium-mediated cellular membrane homeostasis, and energy metabolism (1). Glutamate elevation has been implicated as a marker of both early ischemic and nonischemic secondary brain injury after intraparenchymal hemorrhage (IPH), TBI, and aSAH (4–6).

Glycerol is a lipid-rich neuronal wall constituent whose elevations in microdialysis assays signify cell loss. As a result, glycerol assays have been utilized as a definitive indicator of ongoing secondary brain injury.

NORMATIVE VALUES FOR STANDARD ANALYTES

There is often temporal variability in concentration of the standard electrolytes, in both normal and diseased states. Best interpretations of cerebral microdialysis data require comparison to previous values and, in some instances, comparison to values within the same patient from another probe location. However, general normal values have been established for adult patients monitored with 10-mm long 20-kDa probes, which were perfused at 0.3 µL/min (Table 6.1; 7).

RISKS OF MONITORING

Placement of an invasive microdialysis probe into a patient's brain has the potential for risks that must be weighed against the benefits of monitoring. That considered, reports of complications resulting from probe placement and maintenance are rare. Most reports of catheter-related hemorrhage or infection come from secondary end points of microdialysis trials intended to explore other monitoring parameters and often report no complications. The risk of brain hemorrhage related to placement of a fiber optic intracranial pressure (ICP) monitor has been reported to be 1% or less in various studies (8). Given the smaller caliber and reduced tensile strength of a microdialysis probe, hemorrhagic complications would be expected to be at least as low. Infection rates for microdialysis probes are often hard to estimate. CSF is not typically monitored for infection during use of the probe, and patients often have other factors that present greater risks for meningitis and ventriculitis. Studies of infection rates for non hollow fiber optic ICP probes estimate the cumulative risk of infection at 1% to 2% throughout the duration of monitoring (8).

Microdialysis probes should be placed under strict sterile conditions, which include use of sterile gown, cap, gloves, and mask. While antibiotics are commonly administered prior to placement of a microdialysis catheter, there are no data to support this protocol or the continued use of antibiotics throughout the use of the catheter. Though also not supported by data, it is customary to verify a normal platelet count (platelets > 100,000 K/µL) and coagulation parameters (INR < 1.4) prior to catheter placement.

INDICATIONS AND EVIDENCE FOR CEREBRAL MICRODIALYSIS MONITORING

The most general indication for use of cerebral microdialysis is concern for secondary brain injury in a patient who is critically ill. The literature has more precisely defined those instances where microdialysis monitoring has proven to be predictive and might be beneficial in guiding therapeutic management. The forthcoming recommendations from the Consensus Summary Statement of the International Multidisciplinary Consensus Conference

TABLE 6.1 Normal Concentrations for Standard Microdialysis Analytes Collected at a Perfusion Rate of 0.3 µL/min

Glucose	2 mM
Pyruvate	120 mM
Lactate	2 mM
Lactate:Pyruvate	15–20
Glutamate	10 mM
Glycerol	20–50 mM

on Multimodality Monitoring in Neurocritical Care will improve uniformity regarding the indications and protocols used for cerebral microdialysis.

ANEURYSMAL SUBARACHNOID HEMORRHAGE

The impact and opportunity for secondary brain injury following aSAH make microdialysis and other multimodal monitoring techniques advisable for guidance of therapy. Nearly 20% of all severe-grade aSAH patients suffer secondary infarction, the vast majority of which are clinically silent (9). Despite its poor recognition, the effect of this injury is not benign and carries substantial negative consequences to long-term recovery. Standard hemodynamic and ICP monitoring and achievement of established goals do not prevent all delayed cerebral infarction (DCI). Biochemical distress is common in aSAH patients despite normal ICP and cerebral perfusion pressures (CPP). In one study, ICP and CPP were shown to be abnormal only 20% of the time that poor brain oxygenation or disturbed cerebral metabolism was observed (10). Critical care of aSAH patients is predicated upon the understanding that therapeutic interventions are possible to reverse ischemic risks. Cerebral microdialysis has been shown to reliably predict the onset of ischemia, particularly with enough warning to enable implementation of a variety of interventions directed toward limiting permanent injury. In a prospective study of aSAH patients, LPR elevations of 20% followed by a 20% glycerol rise predicted delayed infarction in 17 of 18 patients (4). The wean warning time was 11 hours previous to infarction. In a similar prospective study, metabolic distress marked by glutamate elevations preceded delayed ischemic events in 87% of patients (11). LPR increase was less frequent (40%), but occurred 17 hours prior to the new deficit. Helbok and colleagues reported that LPR rise in combination with glucose depression were particularly sensitive for ischemic change, especially when the probe was located in the distribution of the ischemic change (9). Less conventional analytes hold promise in heralding ischemic risk. In a comparative study of aSAH patients with (30%) and without symptomatic vasospasm, higher concentrations of glyceraldehyde-3-phosphate dehydrogenase and lower concentrations of heat-shock cognate were predictive of spasm 4 days prior to onset (12).

LPR elevations after aSAH may have multiple sources and are not exclusively attributable to ischemia. If lactate is elevated in the setting of elevated pyruvate and hyperglycolysis, there may be minimal detrimental impact upon clinical outcome. Conversely, when lactate elevations (> 4 mmol/L) are coincident with associated brain hypoxia defined by (partial brain tissue oxygen) $PbtO_2$ < 20 mmHg, chances for good outcome are less likely (13). While ischemia is a predominant mediator of injury after aSAH, Type II LPR changes do occur.

Recent studies have revealed that a portion of delayed infarction after aSAH is not clearly associated with cerebral vasospasm. The electrical phenomenon of spreading depolarizations may explain this phenomenon. Decreases in glucose and increases in lactate concentrations have been correlated with nonischemic spreading depolarizations identified on subdural grids (14). Microdialysis findings have helped to implicate clustering of spreading depolarizations as a risk for delayed ischemic injury.

Literature regarding the impact of hyperglycemia upon ischemic change and the potential harm of tight glycemic control on critically ill patients are conflicting. In the setting of metabolic distress after aSAH, measures to tightly control serum glucose have been shown to lower brain glucose to dangerous levels (15). While there is often poor connection between serum and brain levels, greater correlation is seen in the setting of normal microdialysis LPR values. This finding may prove beneficial for individualization of glycemic control.

As with glycemic control, much attention has been directed toward defining transfusion thresholds to optimize oxygen delivery to the brain after aSAH. Considering the multitude of patient variables affecting optimal cerebral oxygenation and perfusion, it seems ill-advised to try to determine a general transfusion threshold applicable to all patients. Reduced hemoglobin concentrations have been associated with metabolic distress (LPR > 40) described by microdialysis and may serve as a preferable gauge of adequate oxygen delivery (16).

Other markers of secondary injury after aSAH have been described. The consequence of ICP elevations in aSAH patients are reflected by severe metabolic disturbances (17). The impact of fever on LPR elevations has been described and shown to be therapeutically modifiable, irrespective of intracranial hypertension (18). TNFα is elevated after aSAH and correlates with volume of intraventricular hemorrhage (19). Its role in vasospasm prediction is being explored since many hypotheses regarding DCI center on upregulation of inflammatory pathways. Finally, improvement of microdialysis neurochemistry has been demonstrated following interventional treatment of cerebral vasospasm (20). Concerns regarding duration of treatment effect may be addressed by pre- and postintervention monitoring.

The Consensus Conference on the Critical Care Management of Subarachnoid Hemorrhage states that microdialysis is capable of predicting outcome and DCI after aSAH (21). Given its demonstrated sensitivity and broad applicability for a multitude of secondary processes, the use of cerebral microdialysis after aSAH has established value.

TRAUMATIC BRAIN INJURY

The secondary sequelae and prognosis for TBI are well described by cerebral microdialysis techniques. In a study of 223 patients with severe TBI, elevated LPR and glutamate concentrations were predictive of mortality (22). Glycerol levels in the first 72 hours after resuscitation also correlated with death. In another study, Stein and colleagues showed that metabolic crisis persisting beyond the first 72 hours after trauma predicted poor outcome, even among well-resuscitated patients (23). Likewise, elevated glutamate levels (> 20 mmol/L) are associated with survival, particularly when they increase over time or persist at elevated concentrations (24). Among survivors, the percent time of LPR elevation specifically correlates with frontal lobe atrophy after TBI (25). Microdialysis is sensitive to the variability of cerebral perfusion after TBI. During periods of compromised autoregulation, impaired perfusion is more likely to adversely affect pericontusional chemistry compared to radiological normal brain (26). Among mechanisms of secondary injury, intracranial hypertension is a common cause of death after severe TBI. Elevations in LPR and glycerol commonly precede elevated ICP by hours (27). However, interpretation of absolute analyte values may require age adjustment after TBI. Glycerol and glutamate concentrations appear to be elevated in older trauma patients (28). Although predictive, some investigators have suggested that many neurochemical disturbances seen after TBI represent static injury that does not evolve throughout the course of recovery (29). The preponderance of evidence refutes this claim and demonstrates that the brain chemistry is dynamic following injury. The modifiable nature of many of these abnormalities remains debatable.

Contrary to aSAH, elevated LPR after TBI is seldom a marker of ischemia. As a result, these two conditions should not share treatment algorithms nor should the interpretation of microdialysis data be similarly regarded. Concomitant positive emission tomography (PET), $PbtO_2$, and microdialysis monitoring in severe TBI patients suggest that the brain's utilization of lactate as a fuel source may occur in aerobic and well-perfused environments and that elevations in lactate do not necessarily result from anaerobic metabolism. The LPR elevations result from a reduction in pyruvate concentration, which may be related to the hyperglycolytic responses of the astrocyte, necessary for reuptake of glutamate to compensate for reduced glucose availability (25). This has parallel implications to glucose management after aSAH. After TBI, low brain glucose may persist despite seemingly normal serum concentrations. In one study of severely injured patients, over 40% of all cerebral glucose assays were depressed (30). Tight glycemic control has been demonstrated to result in metabolic distress, marked by elevated glutamate and LPR (6). Magnoni and colleagues believe that low brain glucose is noteworthy only when oxidative metabolism is disturbed (LRP > 25). When brain metabolism is homeostatic, better correlations are seen between serologic and brain glucose concentrations (31).

Despite the recognition of LPR Type II distress, enhanced oxygenation may be considered as a therapeutic measure for TBI patients. Normobaric hyperoxia has been shown to improve LPR after TBI (32). It is possible that a higher partial oxygen pressure (PaO_2) is required to drive oxygen into dysfunctional mitochondria, particularly in the early setting of hyperglycolytic metabolic distress.

INTRAPARENCHYMAL HEMORRHAGE

Neurochemical understanding of secondary injury after IPH is less well established than for aSAH and TBI. Perihematomal tissue does not appear to be subject to ischemic injury in the early phase of recovery after hemorrhage (5). Evacuation of blood products results in reduced brain edema and interstitial glutamate, which contrasts the natural evolution for persistent hematomas. In a study by Ko and colleagues, CPP was not as tightly correlated to metabolic distress as it was to regional hypoxia, whereas patients without disordered autoregulation were more likely to have metabolic distress. As a result, metabolic crisis, marked by elevations in LPR, appears to be related to mitochondrial dysfunction as opposed to impaired perfusion (33). Absence of LPR elevations is tied to more favorable recovery after severe IPH (34).

ISCHEMIC STROKE

Compared to other disease processes, secondary injury after ischemic stroke would seem to be the most neurochemically straightforward. However, few microdialysis studies have explored the ischemic risk following acute stroke. Those studies that have been completed sought to assess the risk of malignant edema after large vessel stroke. The decision to pursue a decompressive hemicraniectomy after massive infarction take into consideration the operative morbidity associated with this treatment and the preferential treatment benefit afforded by early intervention. Patterns of neurochemical distress have been categorized that are predictive of progression to malignant edema (35). For these observations to receive greater consideration in surgical planning after ischemic stroke, the findings of these small studies will require validation and prospective examination.

BRAIN TUMORS

Microdialysis is relatively unexplored as a tool to guide acute treatment for patients with brain tumors. The monitor has been used to investigate perioperative changes and chemotherapeutic infiltration of the tumor bed. The time course of change of various cytokines (IL-8, IP-10, MCP-1, MIP-1, IL-6, INRα, G-CSF, VEGF) has been reported after primary and metastatic tumor resection. In general, inflammatory cytokines were progressively decreased over time (36). Marcus and colleagues neurochemically characterized the resection margin of a cohort of high grade primary brain tumors and correlated World Health Organization (WHO) grade with metabolic activity (37).

HEPATIC ENCEPHALOPATHY

Cerebral microdialysis has been anecdotally reported to be helpful in characterization of the mechanisms associated with hepatic encephalopathy as well as guidance of substrate delivery during hepatic failure (38). Assay of interstitial ammonia concentrations are reflective of astrocyte function and have been shown to correlate with ICP. Glutamate and other cerebral amino acid concentrations also mirror ammonia levels.

ANTIBIOTIC CENTRAL NERVOUS SYSTEM PENETRATION AND DRUG DELIVERY

Plasma concentrations of medications routinely provide misleading insight regarding CNS penetration. If expected recovery is known, microdialysis can give real-time feedback regarding extent of drug delivery. The blood–brain barrier is unpredictably disrupted as a result of meningitis, brain tumors, TBI, and IPH. Additionally, commonly used medications may open (mannitol) or close (corticosteroids) this barrier. Vancomycin, meropenem, and doripenem levels have been assayed through microdialysis recovery (2). Brain concentrations of cefotaxime have been shown to be a portion of the serum levels, and the minimum inhibitory concentrations achieved are highly dependent upon adjustment of dosing intervals (39). Anticonvulsant drugs have been assayed by microdialysis to confirm absorption and delivery (5). This approach is especially appealing for cases of refractory status epilepticus. Finally, penetration of chemotherapeutic agents, such as temozolamide and methotrexate, has been explored in glioma patients to assess adequacy of delivery and to allow minimization of systemic side effects.

PEDIATRIC PATIENTS

Microdialysis use in children has been sparse. Many aspects of pediatric physiology should prompt caution against extrapolation of adult data to this group. Children are generally more tolerant of ICP elevations than adults, even after closure of the fontanelles and fusion of the cranial bones. Compared to the focal traumatic lesions of adults, children commonly possess diffuse brain injury and experience less postinjury edema. Finally, the immature brain appears to be more resilient to the effects of hypoxic injury (40). Considering the increased longevity of disability inherent to brain-injured children and their robust capacity for recovery, further exploration into the benefits of monitor-guided therapy appears appropriate.

WHEN AND WHERE MICRODIALYSIS PROBES SHOULD BE PLACED

Cerebral microdialysis is a regional monitor and the information acquired is representative of the brain chemistry within a small distance from the probe tip. Therefore, proper placement of the microdialysis probe is dependent on the type of information sought and the disease process of each patient. After aSAH, patients suffering delayed infarction acquire the new lesion ipsilateral to the site of aneurysm 93% of the time and within the same vascular territory in 86% of cases (41). A monitoring device with ideal sensitivity would detect evidence of delayed infarction in 71% of cases if placed in the middle cerebral artery territory on the same side as the ruptured aneurysm. Infarction resulting from midline aneurysms, such as those arising from the anterior communicating artery, are difficult to predict and probes should be placed in the hemisphere with the greater volume of subarachnoid blood. Injury may be more diffuse after TBI.

Pericontusional tissue has more greatly disordered metabolism than normal-appearing brain (26) and may be more sensitive to variations in cerebral perfusion. Commonly, probes are placed in the frontal lobes near lesions of concern, but away from regions of obvious radiologic damage. Obvious anatomic limitations may limit desired probe placement. Probes should not be placed in the posterior fossa and are seldom placed in hemispheres that have undergone a craniectomy. The trajectory of probe insertion should also not pass through extra-axial hemorrhage. Placement of the probe should be confirmed with a non-contrast head CT.

The timing of catheter placement also depends upon the mechanism of injury. TBI is marked by early dynamic changes in cerebral blood flow in patients with impaired auto-regulation. Furthermore, brain edema and hemorrhagic expansion tend to occur early in the course of injury. Microdialysis probe placement should be considered in an eligible patient as soon as the patient is resuscitated and within hours of the primary injury. After aSAH, the primary concern for secondary injury is usually related to vasospasm-associated ischemia. Since the peak of vasospasm onset is approximately 5 days after hemorrhage (42), microdialysis monitoring should begin on posthemorrhage day 3 or 4 to allow capture of baseline neurochemistry prior to ischemic risk and to optimize probe durability. Probe placement for other conditions should be tailored to the timing of risk for secondary injury or therapeutic value.

DEVELOPING A SYSTEM FOR RESPONSIVE MICRODIALYSIS THERAPEUTIC GUIDANCE

Brain monitoring is most efficacious when the indications and goals of monitoring are well defined and agreed upon in advance of individual patient care. Formulating clearly stated policies and procedures for microdialysis monitoring is the first and most important step in establishing a monitoring program. Examples of eligibility requirements and guidelines directing consideration of microdialysis placement are included (Tables 6.2 and 6.3).

TABLE 6.2 Guidelines for Cerebral Microdialysis Monitoring After Aneurysmal Subarachnoid Hemorrhage (aSAH)

Eligibility for Cerebral Microdialysis Neuromonitoring (cMDNM) after aSAH

1. Patients eligible for cMDNM must be suspected of having suffered an acute aneurysmal hemorrhage and have risk of acquiring injury related to vasospasm, edema, or other secondary processes.

2. Candidates for cMDNM must possess an alteration in consciousness or incapacity to participate in a thorough neurologic examination (Hunt and Hess Grades IV and V) such that clinical deterioration cannot be readily appreciated.

3. Patients requiring sedative therapy for agitation, ICP control, or other medical causes are eligible for cMDNM.

4. Patients who are fully and consistently alert and participatory in the examination process should not undergo invasive cMDNM.

5. Patients with refractory thrombocytopenia (< 100,000 platelets) or irreversible coagulopathy (INR > 1.4) should not have a microdialysis probe placed.

Timing, Location, and Decision for Microdialysis Catheter Placement After aSAH

1. Catheters should be placed at a time that optimally assesses the patient's risk for secondary injury and minimizes the duration of neuromonitoring.

2. Catheter placement should be considered when there is deterioration in the patient's condition that is suspected to be attributable to secondary injury.

3. For patients who are comatose, monitoring should begin on postbleed day 3 to allow for acquisition of baseline data prior to entering into the period of highest vasospasm risk.

4. If possible, catheters should be placed in the hemisphere ipsilateral to the ruptured aneurysm and in the vascular territory of the parent vessel.

5. The duration of neuromonitoring should take into account the duration of vasospasm risk as well as the approved duration of accuracy for the chosen neuromonitoring probe (5–7 days).

6. The decision to place a neuromonitoring device requires both the approval of the neurointensivist and the primary neurosurgeon.

7. Microdialysis probes should be placed only by those individuals with expertise in monitor placement and those with the appropriate procedural competencies.

Cerebral Microdialysis

Interstitial fluid collection and analysis will occur hourly and the neurocritical care team will be made aware of results based upon the following thresholds:

Glucose < 0.5 mmol/L

Glutamate > 12 mmol/L

Lactate/pyruvate > 25

Glycerol > 100 mmol/L

TABLE 6.3 Guidelines for Cerebral Microdialysis Monitoring After Severe Traumatic Brain Injury (TBI)

Eligibility for Cerebral Microdialysis Neuromonitoring (cMDNM) after Severe TBI

1. Patients eligible for cMDNM must have suffered severe TBI and have a post-resuscitation GCS ≤ 8 or possess clinical evidence that a particular region of the brain is at high risk for secondary injury related to vasospasm, edema, or other secondary processes.

2. Patients requiring sedative therapy for agitation, ICP control, or other medical causes are eligible for cMDNM. Patients who are intolerant of regular sedation weaning or unable to have frequent neurologic assessments for another cause should be considered for neuromonitoring.

3. Patients who are fully and consistently alert and participatory in the examination process should not undergo invasive cMDNM.

4. Patients with refractory thrombocytopenia (< 100,000 platelets) or irreversible coagulopathy (INR > 1.4) should not have a microdialysis probe placed.

Timing, Location, and Decision for Microdialysis Catheter Placement After Severe TBI

1. Catheters should be placed early in the course of critical care to optimally assess the patient's risk for secondary injury.

2. Catheter placement should be considered when there is deterioration in the patient's condition that is suspected to be attributable to secondary injury.

3. For patients with diffuse injury or for use of the probe in global brain assessment, the catheter should be placed in the frontal lobe (preferably right) in a brain region devoid of obvious radiological injury.

4. For provision of regional data related to a specific lesion, the catheter should be placed in a peri lesional location with the use of neuronavigational guidance (if necessary).

5. Duration of neuromonitoring should take into account the duration of risk of secondary injury as well as the approved duration of accuracy for the chosen neuromonitoring probe (5–7 days).

6. The decision to place a cMDNM requires both the approval of the neurointensivist and the primary neurosurgeon.

7. Microdialysis catheters should be placed only by those individuals with expertise in monitor placement and those with the appropriate procedural competencies.

Cerebral Microdialysis

Interstitial fluid collection and analysis will occur hourly and the neurocritical care team will be made aware of results based upon the following thresholds:

Glucose < 0.5 mmol/L

Glutamate > 12 mmol/L

Lactate/pyruvate > 25

Glycerol > 100 mmol/L

TABLE 6.4 Checklist to Guide Assessment of Elevated Microdialysis Lactate Pyruvate Ratio and Glutamate Levels

Cerebral Microdialysis Abnormal Analyte Checklist: Elevated LPR and Glutamate
LPR > 25
Glutamate > 12 mmol/L
1. Ensure that microdialysis probe is in viable tissue and that appropriate fluid volume has been recovered from the microvial (18 uL/hr).
2. Verify that patient is not febrile.
3. Evaluate if patient is seizing.

4. For concerns of ischemia:
    A. Can hemoglobin concentration be further optimized?
    B. Ensure that ICP is well controlled.
    C. Optimize CPP to see if neurochemistry can be improved.
    D. Assess for vasospasm—TCD, CTA, catheter angiography.
    E. Verify CO_2 is in range and patient is not pathologically hyperventilated.

5. Optimize hemoglobin saturation:
    A. Increase fraction of inspired oxygen (FiO_2)?
    B. Increase positive end-expiratory pressure (PEEP).
    C. Ensure ventilator synchrony.

6. Assess worsening of brain edema:
    A. Optimize hyperosmolar therapy.
    B. Control fever.
    C. Evaluate for surgical lesion.

Brain metabolism and the neurochemical changes that signal secondary injury occur on a minute to hourly time scale. Integration of microdialysis monitoring into the therapeutic plan requires that a system is in place that immediately alerts the treatment team to neurochemical changes and allows timely implementation of corrective measures. All members of the multidisciplinary team must understand the goals of therapy and be accountable for their role in the detection, decision making, and interventional aspects of monitoring. Expectations for monitoring and uniform approaches to abnormalities are best integrated into monitoring order sets, flow sheets, and checklists. A sample check list (Table 6.4) and flow sheet (Figure 6.2) describing approaches to disordered neurochemistry are provided.

CONCLUSION

In critical care of the brain-injured patient, general hemodynamic guided therapies fail to identify and prevent a substantial portion of secondary injury. Individualization of care is required to tailor therapy to the specific needs of the patient. Cerebral microdialysis provides a wealth of information regarding the health of the injured brain and provides

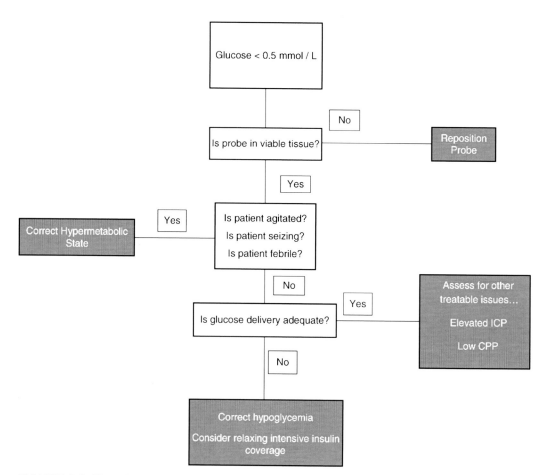

FIGURE 6.2 Flow sheet demonstrating a systematic approach to abnormally low microdialysis glucose concentrations.

preemptive insight into the modifiable mechanisms of delayed disability. The utility of microdialysis is most developed in TBI and aSAH, but the potential for this neuromonitor is largely unexplored.

REFERENCES

1. Larach DB, Kofke WA, and Le Roux P. Potential non-hypoxic/ischemic causes of increased cerebral interstitial fluid lactate/pyruvate ratio: A review of available literature. *Neurocrit Care.* 2011;15:609–622.

2. Shannon RJ, Carpenter KLH, Guilfoyle MR, et al. Cerebral microdialysis in clinical studies of drugs: pharmacokinetic applications. *J Pharmacokinet Pharmacodyn.* 2013;40:343–58.

3. Helmy A, Carpenter KLH, Skeper JN, et al. microdialysis of cytokines: methodological considerations, scanning electron microscopy, and determination of relative recovery. *Journal of Neurotrauma.* 2009;26:549–561.

4. Skjoth-Rasmussen J, Schulz M, Kristensen SR, et al. Delayed neurological deficits detected by an ischemic pattern in the extracellular cerebral metabolites in patients with aneurysmal subarachnoid hemorrhage. *J Neurosurg.* 2004;100:8–15.

5. Miller CM, Vespa PM, McArthur DL, et al. Frameless stereotactic aspiration and thrombolysis of deep intracerebral hemorrhage is associated with reduced levels of extracellular cerebral glutamate and unchanged lactate pyruvate ratios. *Neurocrit Care.* 2007;6:22–29.
6. Vespa P, Boonyaputthikul R, McArthur DL, et al. Intensive insulin therapy reduces microdialysis glucose values without altering glucose utilization or improving the lactate/pyruvate ratio after traumatic brain injury. *Crit Care Med.* 2006;34:850–856.
7. Schulz MK, Wang LP, Tange M, et al. Cerebral microdialysis monitoring: determination of normal and ischemic cerebral metabolism in patients with aneurysmal subarachnoid hemorrhage. *J Neurosurg.* 2000;93(5):808–814.
8. Bekar A, Dogan S, Abas F, et al. Risk factors and complications of intracranial pressure monitoring with a fiberoptic device. *J of Clin Neuroscience.* 2009;16(2):236–240.
9. Helbok R, Madineni RC, Schmidt MJ, et al. Intracerebral monitoring of silent infarcts after subarachnoid hemorrhage. *Neurocrit Care.* 2011;14:162–167.
10. Chen HI, Steifel MF, Oddo M, et al. Detection of cerebral compromise with multimodality monitoring in patients with subarachnoid hemorrhage. *Neurosurgery.* 2011;69:53–63.
11. Samuelsson C, Hillered L, Enblad P, et al. Microdialysis patterns in subarachnoid hemorrhage patients with focus on ischemic events and brain interstitial glutamine levels. *Acta Neurochir.* 2009;151:437–446.
12. Maurer MH, Haux D, Sakowitz OW, et al. Identification of early markers for symptomatic vasospasm in human cerebral microdialysate after subarachnoid hemorrhage: Preliminary results of a proteome-wide screening. *Journal of Cerebral Blood Flow and Metabolism.* 2007;27:1675–1683.
13. Oddo M, Levine JM, Frangos S, et al. Brain lactate metabolism in humans with subarachnoid hemorrhage. *Stroke.* 2012;43:1418–1421.
14. Sakowitz OW, Santos E, Nagel A, et al. Clusters of spreading depolarizations are associated with disturbed cerebral metabolism in patients with aneurysmal subarachnoid hemorrhage. *Stroke.* 2013;44:220–223.
15. Schmidt JM, Claassen J, Ko S, et al. Nutritional support and brain tissue glucose metabolism in poor-grade SAH: a retrospective observational study. *Critical Care.* 2012;16:R15.
16. Kurtz P, Schmidt JM, Claassen J, et al. Anemia is associated with metabolic distress and brain tissue hypoxia after subarachnoid hemorrhage. *Neurocrit Care.* 2010;13:10–16.
17. Nagel A, Graetz D, Schink T, et al. Relevance of intracranial hypertension for cerebral metabolism in aneurysmal subarachnoid hemorrhage. *J Neurosurg.* 2009;111:94–101.
18. Oddo M, Frangos S, Milby A, et al. Induced normothermia attenuates cerebral metabolic distress in patients with aneurysmal subarachnoid hemorrhage and refractory fever. *Stroke.* 2009;40:1913–1916.
19. Hanafy KA, Grobelny B, Fernandez L, et al. Brain interstitial fluid TNF-α after subarachnoid hemorrhage. *J of Neurological Sciences.* 2010;291:69–73.
20. Stuart RM, Helbok R, Kurtz, et al. High-Dose Intra-arterial verapamil for the treatment of cerebral vasospasm after subarachnoid hemorrhage: Prolonged effects on hemodynamic parameters and brain metabolism. *Neurosurgery.* 2011;68:337–345.
21. Hanggi D, and The participants in the International Multi-disciplinary Consensus Conference on the Critical Care Management of Subarachnoid Hemorrhage. *Neurocrit Care.* 2011;15:318–323.
22. Timofeev I, Carpenter KLH, Nortje J, et al. Cerebral extracellular chemistry and outcome following traumatic brain injury: a microdialysis study of 223 patients. *Brain.* 2011;134:484–494.
23. Stein NR, McArthur DL, Etchepare M, et al. Early cerebral metabolic crisis after TBI influences outcome despite adequate hemodynamic resuscitation. *Neurocrit Care.* 2012;17:49–57.
24. Chamoun R, Suki D, Gopinath SP, et al. Role of extracellular glutamate measured by cerebral microdialysis in severe traumatic brain injury. *J Neurosurg.* 2010;113:564–570.
25. Marcoux J, McArthur DA, Miller C, et al. Persistent metabolic crisis as measured by elevated cerebral microdialysis lactate-pyruvate ratio predicts chronic frontal lobe brain atrophy after traumatic brain injury. *Crit Care Med.* 2008;36:2871–2877.
26. Timofeev I, Czosnyka M, Carpenter KLH, et al. Interaction between brain chemistry and physiology after traumatic brain injury: Impact of autoregulation and microdialysis catheter location. *Journal of Neurotrauma.* 2011;28:849–860.

27. Adamides AA, Rosenfeldt FL, Winter CD, et al. Brain tissue lactate elevations predict episodes of intracranial hypertension in patients with traumatic brain injury. *J Am Coll Surg.* 2009;209(4):531–539.
28. Mellergard P, Sjogren F, and Hillman J. The cerebral extracellular release of glycerol, glutamate, and FGF2 is increased in older patients following severe traumatic brain injury. *Journal of Neurotrauma.* 2012;29:112–118.
29. Nelson DW, Thornquist B, MacCallum RM, et al. Analysis of cerebral microdialysis in patients with traumatic brain injury: relations to intracranial pressure, cerebral perfusion pressure and catheter placement. *BMC Medicine.* 2011;9:21.
30. Oddo M, Schmidt JM, Carrera E, et al. Impact of tight glycemic control on cerebral glucose metabolism after severe brain injury: A microdialysis study. *Crit Care Med.* 2008;36:3233–3238.
31. Magnoni S, Tedesco C, Carbonara M, et al. Relationship between systemic glucose and cerebral glucose is preserved in patients with severe traumatic brain injury, but glucose delivery to the brain may become limited when oxidative metabolism is impaired: Implications for glycemic control. *Crit Care Med.* 2012;40:1785–1791.
32. Tisdall MM, Tachtsidis I, Leung TS, et al. Increase in cerebral aerobic metabolism by normobaric hyperoxia after traumatic brain injury. *J Neurosurg.* 2008;109:424–432.
33. Ko S, Choi HA, Parikh G, et al. Multimodality monitoring for cerebral perfusion optimization in comatose patients with intracerebral hemorrhage. *Stroke.* 2011;42:3087–3092.
34. Nikaina I, Paterakis K, Paraforos G, et al. Cerebral perfusion pressure, microdialysis biochemistry, and clinical outcome in patients with spontaneous intracerebral hematomas. *Journal of Critical Care.* 2012;27:83–88.
35. Schnewies S, Grond M, Staub F, et al. Predictive value of neurochemical monitoring in large middle cerebral artery infarction. *Stroke.* 2001;32:1863–1867.
36. Portnow J, Badie B, Liu X, et al. A pilot microdialysis study in brain tumor patients to assess changes in intracerebral cytokine levels after craniotomy and in response to treatment with a targeted anti-cancer agent. *J Neurooncol.* 2013; e-pub before print.
37. Marcus HJ, Carpenter KLH, Price SJ, et al. In vivo assessment of high-grade glioma biochemistry using microdialysis: A study of energy-related molecules, growth factors and cytokines. *J Neurooncol.* 2010;97:11–23.
38. Rivera-Espinosa L, Floriano-Sanchez E, Pedraza-Chaverri J, et al. Contributions of Microdialysis to New Alternative Therapeutics for Hepatic Encephalopathy. *Int. J. Mol. Sci.* 2013;14:16184–16206.
39. Dahyot-Fizelier C, Frasca D, Gregoire N, et al. Microdialysis study of cefotaxime cerebral distribution in patients with acute brain injury. *Antimicrob. Agents Chemother.* 2013;57(6):2738.
40. Charalambides C, Sgouros, and Sakas D. Intracerebral microdialysis in children. *Childs Nerv Syst.* 2010;26:215–220.
41. Miller CM and Palestrant D. Distribution of delayed ischemic neurological deficits after aneurysmal subarachnoid hemorrhage and implications for regional neuromonitoring. *Clinical Neurology and Neurosurgery.* 2012;114:545–549.
42. Miller CM, Palestrant D, Schievink WI, et al. Prolonged Transcranial Doppler Monitoring After Aneurysmal Subarachnoid Hemorrhage Fails to Adequately Predict Ischemic Risk. *Neurocrit Care.* 2011;15:387–392.

Cerebral Autoregulation

Marek Czosnyka, PhD
Enrique Carrero Cardenal, PhD

INTRODUCTION

Patients with brain injuries may have impaired cerebral autoregulation.

The extent of this impairment may fluctuate with time. A repeatable noninvasive method of monitoring of autoregulatory reserve is needed.

If autoregulation is altered, it decreases the range of cerebral perfusion pressure (CPP) that ensures adequate cerebral blood flow (CBF) as it becomes pressure passive. The risk of cerebral hypoperfusion ischemia (1,2), or hyperemia, edema, and cerebral bleeding increases (3). Patients with severe brain injury and impaired cerebral autoregulation have poor outcome (4).

Several modalities are frequently used for monitoring cerebral autoregulation. They are reviewed, along with comprehensive assessment of soundness of the reported results.

TRANSCRANIAL DOPPLER ULTRASONOGRAPHY

Transcranial Doppler (TCD) ultrasonography has the ability to continuously assess the autoregulatory reserve.

The versatility of TCD has encouraged imaginative applications in head-injured patients, allowing both dynamic and static tests to be evaluated in the clinical setting (5–7).

Static Test of Autoregulation

Methods for the static assessment of autoregulation rely on observing middle cerebral artery (MCA) blood flow velocity (FV) during changes in mean arterial blood pressure (ABP) induced by an infusion of vasopressor (Figure 7.1). The static rate of autoregulation (SRoR) can be calculated as the percentage increase in vascular resistance divided by the percentage rise in CPP (8). A SRoR of 100% indicates perfect functionality, whereas a SRoR of 0% indicates fully depleted autoregulation. The test is potentially prone to

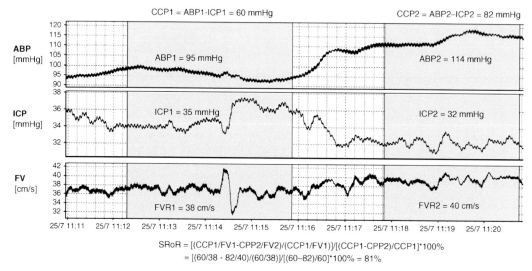

FIGURE 7.1 Example of measurement of SRoR in a TBI patient. ABP has been raised with norepinephrine. Baseline values (index 1) were compared with values recorded after elevation of ABP by 19 mmHg (index 2). SRoR has been calculated as relative increase in CVR (CPP/FV, where FV was mean blood FV in the MCA and CPP) divided by relative increase in CPP (see formula under the graph). In this particular case SRoR revealed properly functioning autoregulation.

overestimation of the autoregulatory reserve caused by the phenomenon of false autoregulation, when only changes in arterial pressure (not CPP) are used for the calculation (9).

Transcranial Doppler Reactivity to Changes in Carbon Dioxide Concentration (10)

Testing for CO_2 cerebrovascular reactivity has been shown to have an important application in the assessment of severely head-injured patients as well as other cerebrovascular diseases. Although many authors have demonstrated that cerebral vessels are reactive to changes in CO_2 when cerebral autoregulation had been already impaired (11). CO_2 reactivity correlates significantly with outcome following head injury (11–13). The test is simple and repeatable. However, in patients with exhausted cerebral compensatory reserve, hypercapnia may provoke substantial changes in intracranial pressure (ICP) (14,15). Therefore, this method cannot be used without consideration of patient safety, particularly if baseline ICP is already elevated. Brief induction of mild hypocapnia (above 4.5 kPa or 34 mmHg) is safer than induction of hypercapnia (Figure 7.2; 16). Also, changes in mean arterial pressure (MAP), induced by change in $PaCO_2$, should be accounted for while calculating reactivity (17). Normal reactivity should stay above 15% per kPa (7.5 mmHg) change in $PaCO_2$.

Thigh Cuff Test

Aaslid described a method in which a step-wise decrease in ABP was achieved by the deflation of compressed leg cuffs while simultaneously measuring TCD FV in the MCA (Figure 7.3; 18). An index, called the dynamic rate of autoregulation (RoR), describes how quickly cerebral vessels react to the sudden fall in blood pressure. The RoR was proposed

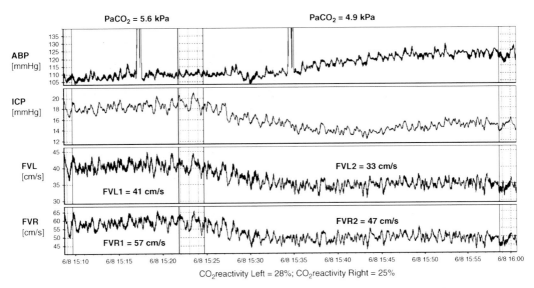

FIGURE 7.2 Example of measurement of CO_2 reactivity in a TBI patient. $PaCO_2$ was decreased to a level of mild hypocapnia by increasing FiO_2. Decrease in mean FV and a slight decrease in ICP were noted. Calculated CO_2 reactivity was very good at both sides (above 20%/kPa).

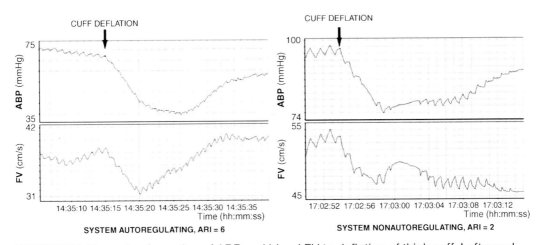

FIGURE 7.3 Example of reaction of ABP and blood FV to deflation of thigh cuff. Left panel shows the scenario of functional autoregulation (index of autoregulation = 6): When following decrease in ABP the flow velocity first decreased but compensatory (autoregulation-mediated) rise was seen very soon. Deteriorated autoregulation is presented in the right panel: With thanks to Prof. L. Steiner. An initial decrease in flow velocity was sustained (ARI = 3).

to express the autoregulatory reserve, and was subsequently shown to correlate with blood CO_2 concentration in volunteers and with static rate of autoregulation. Index of autoregulation (ARI) (graded from 0–impaired autoregulation, to 9–intact autoregulation) was introduced by Tiecks and colleagues (19). In clinical practice, a potentially confounding factor may result from neglecting the changes in ICP, since this varies with rapid changes in arterial pressure according to the state of the cerebral autoregulation (20–22).

Transient Hyperaemic Response Test

Short-term compression of the common carotid artery (CCA) produces a marked decrease in the MCA blood FV in the ipsilateral hemisphere. During compression, the distal cerebrovascular bed dilates if autoregulation is intact. Upon release of the compression, a transient hyperaemia, lasting for few seconds, occurs until the distal cerebrovascular bed constricts to its former diameter. This indicates a positive autoregulatory response (Figure 7.4; 23–25). The test was introduced in the late 1980s and can be used in the assessment of a number of different cerebral conditions, including head injury (26) and subarachnoid hemorrhage (27). However, results depend on the technique of compression (23,25) and, in patients with carotid disease, there are theoretical risks associated with the maneuver (28). In head-injured patients, variations in ICP following compression of the CCA are possible (29). The clinical results showed a positive correlation between the presence of a hyperaemic response and outcome following head injury (26).

Phase Shift Between Transcranial Doppler and Mean Arterial Pressure During Slow Respiration

An interesting method of deriving the autoregulatory status from natural fluctuations in MCA flow velocity involves the assessment of phase shift between the superimposed respiratory and ABP waves during slow (6 per minute) breathing. A 0° phase shift indicates absent autoregulation, whereas a phase shift of 90° or more indicates intact autoregulation. This method has not been formally applied to the analysis of TCD waveform in head-injured patients. However, it is attractive since the respiratory waveform can be investigated safely and repeated with ease. Such an approach may allow for the continuous assessment of autoregulation without performing potentially hazardous provocative maneuvers on arterial pressure (30–34).

Correlation Method Using Transcranial Doppler Flow Velocity Waveform

Experimental and modeling studies demonstrate the specific patterns of the stable systolic and falling diastolic values of pulsatile pattern in FV when CPP decreases during

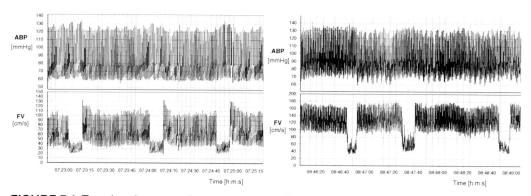

FIGURE 7.4 Transient hyperaemic response test. Following occlusion of the carotid artery, hyperaemia is seen in autoregulating patient (left panel). No hyperaemia is seen in the patient with depleted autoregulation (right panel).

controlled hemorrhage or intracranial hypertension (35–37). When CPP decreases, cortical blood flow only starts to decrease when both the systolic and diastolic FV are decreasing. With CPP monitored continuously in severely head-injured patients, correlation coefficients, between consecutive samples of the averaged (10 seconds window) CPP and the different components of the FV (systolic FV, mean FV), were calculated over 5-minute epochs, and then averaged for each patient. These correlation coefficients were named, respectively, systolic (Sx) and mean (Mx) indices. The signs (+ve or –ve) of the correlation coefficients may be interpreted as directions of the regression lines describing the relationships between the systolic FV and mean FV versus CPP (Figure 7.5). A positive correlation coefficient signifies positive association of FV with CPP absent autoregulation. A negative correlation coefficient signifies a negative association—that is, autoregulation present. Correlation coefficients are more suitable for comparison between patients than the regression gradients themselves, as they have standardized values from –1 to +1.

Group analyses demonstrated that clinical outcome following head injury was dependent on the averaged autoregulation indices. Time analysis demonstrated that autoregulation was most likely to be compromised during the first 2 days after admission for those patients with a fatal outcome (38,39).

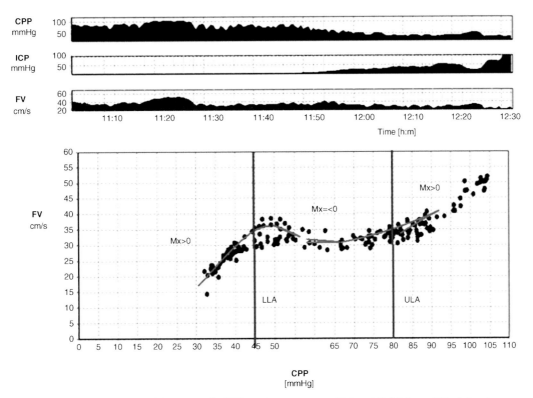

FIGURE 7.5 Experimental increase in ICP and response of blood FV. Mean FV plotted versus CPP (lower panel) shows Lassen curve with lower and upper limit of autoregulation. Within the autoregulation range, the correlation between slow changes in CPP and FV is zero or negative (zero or negative Mx), outside positive (positive Mx) (upper panel).

Transfer Function Analysis

This method uses modeling of the step response of the system generating changes of FV from changes in ABP. For assessment of autoregulation based on spontaneous fluctuations of ABP, values of autoregulation index (ARI) are obtained by fitting the second-order linear model proposed by Tiecks et al (19) describing the FV response to the step-change in ABP. Transfer function analysis is used to quantify the dynamic relationship between mean ABP (input) and mean FV (output). The inverse Fourier transform is then performed to obtain the FV impulse response in time domain. Impulse response is, in turn, integrated to yield an estimate of the FV response to a hypothetical step change in ABP. Each of the 10 models, corresponding to ARI values from 0 (absence of autoregulation) to 9 (best autoregulation), is fitted to the first 10 seconds of the FV step response. The best fit, as selected by the minimum squared error, is taken as the representative value of ARI for that segment of data. ARI proved to correlate with outcome following TBI (39,40–42). Threshold ARI (although autoregulation is not an all-or-nothing phenomenon) is around 3 to 4. ARI, similar to Mx, is suitable to monitor autoregulation continuously during dynamical processes like plateau waves of ICP (Figure 7.6).

INTRACRANIAL PRESSURE AND ARTERIAL BLOOD PRESSURE

Brain-injured, critically ill patients on mechanical ventilation exhibit slow (20 seconds to 3 min) ABP variations leading to quantifiable cerebrovascular vasomotor responses. Czosnyka et al (43) studied 83 severe TBI patients using in-house software analysis of on-line physiologic data to collect and calculate time-averaged values of ICP, ABP, and CPP (the authors used waveform time integration for 10-sec intervals). Linear (Pearson's) moving correlation coefficients between 30 past consecutive 10-second averages of ICP and ABP, designated as the pressure-reactivity index (PRx), were computed. A positive PRx signifies a positive association (ie, positive gradient of the regression line) between the slow components of ABP and ICP, indicating a passive nonreactive behavior of the vascular bed. A negative value of PRx reflects a normally reactive vascular bed, with ABP waves provoking inversely correlated waves in ICP (Figure 7.7). Because the correlation

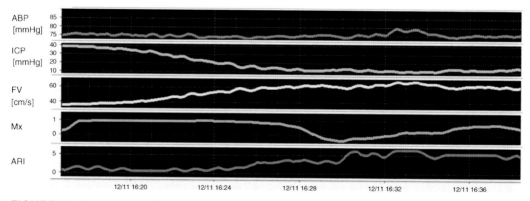

FIGURE 7.6 Transfer function analysis during trailing edge of ICP plateau wave (ICP decreasing from 40 to 15 mmHg). Both ARI (increasing) and Mx (decreasing) indicated improving cerebral autoregulation seen after plateau wave. Thanks to "Mary" Xiuyun Liu.

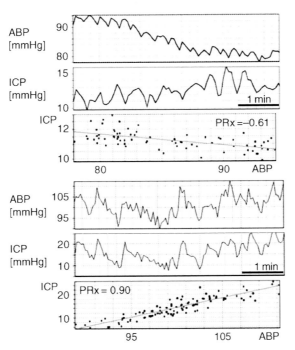

FIGURE 7.7 PRx as correlation coefficient between slow changes in ABP and ICP (30 consecutive mean 10 sec values of both signals). Negative PRx indicates good cerebrovascular reactivity (upper panel) and positive-deteriorated reactivity (lower panel). Illustration courtesy of Dr. Andrea Lavinio.

coefficient has a standardized value (range −1 to +1), PRx provides a convenient index, suitable for comparison among patients. A positive PRx correlated significantly with high ICP, low admission Glasgow Coma Scale (GCS) score, and poor outcome at 6 months after injury. The correlation between PRx and TCD-derived index of autoregulation was highly significant.

The PRx may be presented and analyzed as a time-dependent variable, responding to dynamic events such as ICP plateau waves or incidents of arterial hypo- and hypertension or refractory intracranial hypertension. Alternatively, PRx may be interpreted as a product of module of coherence between ABP and ICP functions in a frequency of slow waves (20 seconds to 3 minutes) multiplied by a cosine of phase shift between ABP and ICP slow waves. Zero-degree phase shift characterizes pressure-passive behavior of vascular walls (PRx = +1, if the coherence is high), whereas a 180-degree phase shift indicates ideally active vasomotor responses (PRx = −1; 44).

The PRx has been validated against a PET-derived static measure of autoregulation (45). Pressure reactivity index and $SRoR_{PET}$ were shown to correlate closely under conditions of disturbed pressure autoregulation. The relationship of PRx with CBF and cerebral metabolic rate for oxygen ($CMRO_2$) was explored in a group of severe TBI patients (46). An inverse relationship between PRx and $CMRO_2$ was found. The data relating the oxygen extraction fraction (OEF) and the PRx followed a quadratic function with disturbed PRx for both low and high OEF. These investigations show that compromised pressure-flow autoregulation, cerebral dysoxia, and metabolic failure are all features of severe TBI and seem to be related at different levels. Yet, we do not currently have a satisfactory mechanistic model that links them.

Timofeev et al (47) correlated brain tissue oxygenation, microdialysis and PRx data from normal and pericontusional brain tissue. Perilesional tissue chemistry exhibited a significant independent relationship with ICP, PbtO$_2$ (brain tissue oxygenation), and CPP thresholds, with increasing lactate/pyruvate (LP) ratio in response to decrease in PbtO$_2$ and CPP, and increase in ICP. The relationship between CPP and chemistry depended upon the state of PRx.

The most important use of PRx is as a time-varying index of autoregulation—see the example in Figure 7.8. In this example, elevated, but stable, ICP was followed by six plateau waves, where PRx reached values close to +1, leading to sustained refractory rise in ICP with PRx permanently elevated.

Optimal CPP

The concept of optimal CPP has been adopted from earlier research (39,48), indicating that many direct and indirect outcome measures or descriptors of autoregulation present with a

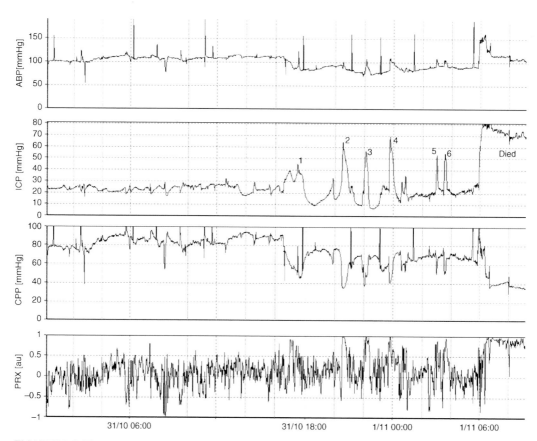

FIGURE 7.8 Time-related changes in ICP, CPP, PRx in a patient who had elevated though stable ICP. After ICP elevations (plateau waves), the patient then developed sudden refractory hypertension and died. During plateau waves (numbered) and refractory hypertension, PRx dynamically increased to values close to +1.

U-shape curve when plotted against CPP. This U shape suggests that, at too low CPP and too high CPP, brain homeostasis becomes compromised. In 2002, Steiner et al (49) published a landmark study on the use of PRx as a means of identifying patient-specific, optimal CPP in long-term ICP/ABP monitoring after TBI. This was a retrospective analysis of prospectively collected data from 114 severe TBI patients receiving intensive care and continuous multimodality monitoring. An optimal CPP (CPP_{opt}) was defined as the CPP range (bins of 5 mmHg) corresponding to the lowest PRx value observed (the lowest or more negative the PRx, the better preserved pressure reactivity is considered to be) (Figure 7.9). Then, the difference between actual mean CPP and CPP_{opt} was calculated and shown to significantly correlate with 6-month outcome. The outcome correlated with this difference for patients who were managed on average below CPP_{opt} and for patients whose mean CPP was above CPP_{opt}. This finding enforces the concept of inappropriate perfusion pressures (on both sides of the spectrum) and their impact on effectiveness of pressure reactivity and clinical outcomes as initially shown by Overgaard and Tweed (50). Another important aspect is the demonstration of the dynamic nature of pressure autoregulation across and within patients, pointing against an "all or nothing" phenomenon. This provides a strong physiologic rationale for individualizing therapy. An important methodological limitation of this study was the fact that, despite obtaining CPP_{opt} for the majority of patients, there were 40% of the cohort where identification of CPP_{opt} was not possible. The authors speculated a number of reasons for failure in these patients, including a CPP_{opt} lying outside of the studied range, inadequate time window and/or data points, and disturbed pressure reactivity for a different etiology than inappropriate CPP. Finally, Steiner et al, based on their findings, proposed an algorithmic approach to identifying CPP_{opt}, setting the stage for a PRx-targeted prospective trial (which has never been conducted). Newer material has been retrospectively studied

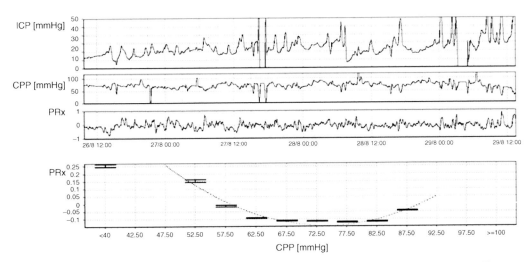

FIGURE 7.9 Optimal CPP curve is a distribution of mean PRx versus observed CPP. Too low CPP indicates ischemia, due to falling CPP and deteriorating reactivity (positive PRx). Too high CPP indicates hyperaemia due to autoregulatory failure at high perfusion pressure (system works predominantly above upper limit of autoregulation). In between, the PRx reaches minimum, which indicates level of optimal CPP at 72 mmHg.

by Aries et al. (51), who analyzed long-term monitoring of ICP and ABP after TBI using a homogeneous software approach at Addenbrooke's Hospital, Cambridge (ICM+: www.neurosurg.cam.ac.uk/icmplus). The algorithm has been improved, incorporating automatic U-shape curves fitting a 4-hour-long moving window. Results tested the early hypothesis of Steiner (49). Optimal CPP can be calculated continuously more than 80% of time and presented as a dynamically changing variable. Continuous metrics of the distance between CPP_{opt} and current CPP relate to outcome. For CPP too low in comparison to CPP_{opt}, mortality dramatically increases. For CPPs too high, incidence of severe disability increases. Favorable outcome reaches its peak if CPP is maintained around CPP_{opt}.

The value of CPP_{opt} has also been recently demonstrated in a pediatric group of TBI patients, where it was significantly associated with survival (52). Pressure-reactivity was found to improve with increasing CPP. The PRx was found to be CPP dependent. The PRx could play a role in assisting determination, not only patient-specific, but also age-specific CPP_{opt} targets.

The concept of "optimal CPP" therapy has never been tried prospectively in a randomized manner. Comparisons between historical groups ($N = 40$), managed with a CPP-oriented protocol, and "autoregulation-oriented therapy," including calculating and following CPP_{opt} ($N = 40$), has been recently presented by the Neurosurgical Burdenko Institute in Moscow (53). They showed significantly better outcomes in the optimal CPP group (median: moderate disability vs. severe disability; $P = .0014$).

BRAIN TISSUE OXYGENATION REACTIVITY

Invasive probes have been developed to monitor focal brain tissue oxygen tension ($PbtO_2$) and represent the balance between oxygen delivery and cellular oxygen consumption (54–56). Its value can be interpreted as a surrogate of the local CBF, but its measurement is influenced by the distance of the tip of the probe to the capillary bed (57). $PbtO_2$ probes provide a highly focal measurement and normal values are in the range of 35 to 50 mmHg. It has been demonstrated that reduced $PbtO_2$ values, and the extent of their duration, are associated with poor outcome after TBI (58–60). The threshold below 15 mmHg is considered high risk, and values below 10 mmHg are associated with irreversible ischemia. A clinical intervention can usually alter $PbtO_2$. Whether the manipulation of this variable can affect outcome is not clear. Just two studies so far could have shown that $PbtO_2$ measurement reduces mortality rate in TBI (61,62).

Fast changes in brain tissue oxygen tension reflect mainly changes in local CBF (providing $CMRO_2$, arterial saturation, and oxygen diffusivity are stable). Therefore, its value can be used to create an ARI similar to Mx or PRx. The oxygen reactivity index (ORx) is the moving correlation coefficient between $PbtO_2$ and CPP. As $PbtO_2$ values are obtained every 30 seconds, the moving correlation window should, accordingly, be at least 30 min to 1 hr. In an experimental clinical study of 14 TBI patients, cerebral tissue oxygen reactivity correlated significantly with the static rate of cerebral autoregulation (63). In this context, a correlation between ORx and PRx was also reported in a study of 27 patients with TBI (46). In regard to clinical outcome, the value of ORx hasn't been clearly elucidated as with Mx or PRx. The patient numbers in the above-mentioned studies were rather small. Jaeger et al (64) could demonstrate an association of ORx and Glasgow Coma Scale (GCS), whereas Radolovich et al (65) could not. Two studies with patients after subarachnoid hemorrhage showed that ORx was independently associated with the occurrence of delayed cerebral infarction (66) and unfavorable outcome (67).

ORx and PRx often present with U-shape type distribution versus CPP. CPP_{opt} for ORx sometimes matches CPP_{opt} for PRx (Figure 7.10); however, overall statistical results are not encouraging (65).

NEAR-INFRARED SPECTROSCOPY

Near-infrared spectroscopy (NIRS; 68,69) was introduced in the 1970s as a technique that was capable of noninvasive monitoring of oxygenation in living tissue based on the transmission and absorption of near-infrared light (700–1,000 nm). Cerebral oxygenation can be determined by the relative absorption of oxygenated and deoxygenated hemoglobin as they have different absorption spectra. The ratio of oxygenated hemoglobin to total hemoglobin and its corresponding percentage value is expressed as the Tissue Oxygenation Index (TOI). The TOI is not a universal fixed term, as different manufacturers of NIRS machines exist and call their indexes differently (eg, rSO_2, CO).

Similar to $PbtiO_2$, the TOI can be regarded as surrogate of changes in local CBF under the assumption that hematocrit, arterial oxygen saturation, and cerebral metabolism remain constant. The modern NIRS machine is able to detect spontaneous low-frequency oscillations (slow waves), which can be used for continuous cerebral autoregulation assessment

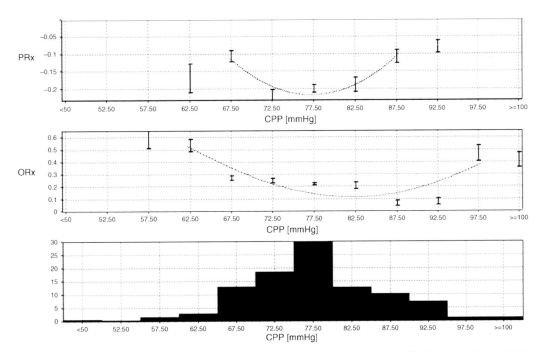

FIGURE 7.10 ORx and PRx sometimes present with similar, U-shape distribution along CPP values. Optimal CPP assessed with ORx (82 mmHg) and PRx (77 mmHg) may vary, but generally stay correlated with each other.

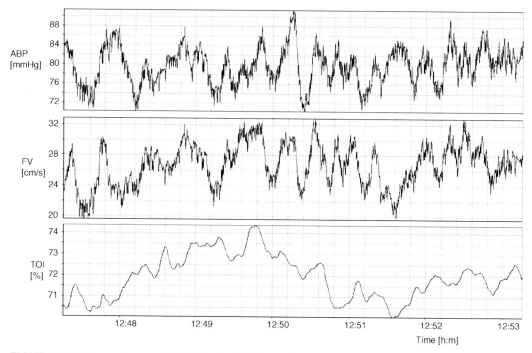

FIGURE 7.11 Recordings of NIRS-derived TOI and TCD blood FV. Slow waves of FV, used for calculation of Mx of autoregulation, are coherent with slow waves of TOI. Therefore, TOI can be also used for continuous monitoring of autoregulation using TOx.

(Figure 7.11). The great advantage of NIRS for cerebral autoregulation monitoring is that this technology is noninvasive. In contrast to TCD, it is very easy to apply. The NIRS sensors are attached to the forehead with self-adhesive pads and do not require frequent calibration, thus making NIRS very suitable for long-term monitoring. It has been demonstrated in a piglet model using controlled reduction of ABP that autoregulation indices derived from NIRS and from cortical blood flow using laser Doppler flowmetry were significantly correlated, and that it was possible to reliably detect the lower limit of autoregulation (70). A high coherence of slow wave fluctuations of TCD-FV and NIRS-TOI signals in the slow wave spectrum was found in a clinical study of sepsis patients (71) and this led to the definition of TOx (other authors also call it COx), which is the moving correlation coefficient between slow waves in TOI and CPP. TOx and TOxa (moving correlation coefficient between ABP and TOI) are significantly correlated to Mx. TOx can be used for optimization of CPP, similar to PRx (Figure 7.12).

The application of NIRS autoregulation monitoring is not just limited to neurocritical care patients. During cardiopulmonary bypass surgery, ABP is empirically managed to targets of putative normal range of cerebral autoregulation. As episodes of hypotension can be very dangerous in such patients, it is preferable that ABP is set individually to a level where autoregulation is intact (72,73). Studies in adults (74) and in children (75) undergoing cardiopulmonary bypass surgery have shown that a NIRS-derived autoregulation index is able to detect dangerous phases of hypotension.

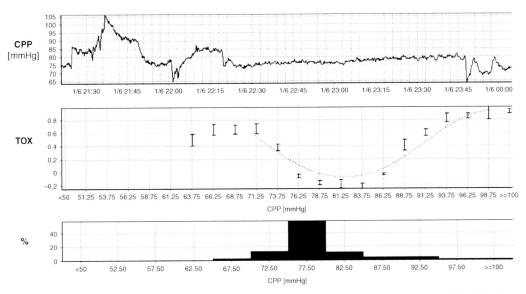

FIGURE 7.12 TOx, distributed along varying CPP, can be used for assessment of optimal CPP (compare to Figure 7.9).

Whereas cerebral autoregulation can be demonstrated by correlation between slow waves of CPP and a surrogate of CBF, vascular reactivity assesses the effect of changes in ABP on a surrogate that measures cerebral blood volume (CBV). NIRS Total Hemoglobin Index (THI) showed a high coherence with slow waves of ICP. A moving correlation coefficient between ABP and THI, called THx (or HVx) correlated significantly with PRx (76,77). An equivalent of THx was also able to detect the lower limit of cerebral autoregulation in an experimental piglet model (76) and impaired cerebrovascular pressure reactivity in TBI patients (defined PRx < 0.3) (78). Because the correlation between the two indices was inconsistent in the latter study, it was aimed to identify situations in which THx is most likely a noninvasive PRx. The results suggested that the agreement between the PRx and THx is a function of the power of slow oscillations in the input signals. This finding confirmed the intuitive notion that adequate assessment of cerebrovascular reactivity in general depends on the occurrence and power of slow wave oscillations. It has been suggested that approximately 50% of the monitoring data would have been rejected because of the absence of sufficient slow wave power. Nevertheless, even without filtering the data for slow wave power, it was possible to determine the optimal CPP and ABP in about 50% of the recordings using THx (77). In the clinical scenario where ICP monitoring is not available, use of THx is appealing for the purpose of optimizing ABP. Regardless, the average bias between PRx- and THx-assessed CPP_{opt} was ± 4.5 mmHg and ± 4.06 mmHg for optimal ABP in the recordings where a direct comparison was possible. The clinical application for optimizing ABP noninvasively would be suited for use in patients in whom invasive ICP monitoring is not possible (79). A noninvasive assessment of a NIRS-based cerebrovascular reactivity index could be a tool to fill the gap between clinical observation alone and invasive ICP monitoring. An example of clinical integration of THx, or HVx, respectively, has been given in a pediatric case with very low birth weight (80). This case report of a critically ill neonate illustrated the potential use of dynamic cerebrovascular reactivity monitoring to detect an impairment prior to the occurrence of intracranial hemorrhage. This case report also pointed out that a NIRS-based index of CBV, such as THx, is probably more robust than CBF-based indices such as TOx or TOxa, as changes in hemoglobin saturations heavily affects TOx/TOxa readings.

CONCLUSION

The main goal of neuromonitoring in patients with brain injury is detecting early risk situations for secondary brain injury.

The neuromonitoring of patients with brain injury must be multimodal. Each monitor reports on a particular aspect of brain injury. The information from the different monitors complement each other and help the clinician to have a more precise idea of the evolving brain injury and how it responds to changes in treatment. Continuous monitoring of cerebral autoregulation is feasible in neurocritical care. In patients with brain injury, conservation of cerebral autoregulation is related to prognosis. Monitoring of cerebral autoregulation is useful for optimizing and individualizing the therapeutic management of patients with brain injury.

Specific assumptions for autoregulation-oriented therapy need to be formulated. It remains to be demonstrated whether this new approach influences patient morbidity and mortality.

REFERENCES

1. Budohoski KP, Czosnyka M, Smielewski P, et al. Impairment of cerebral autoregulation predicts delayed cerebral ischemia after subarachnoid hemorrhage: a prospective observational study. *Stroke.* 2012;43(12):3230–3237.
2. Reinhard M, Rutsch S, Lambeck J, et al. Dynamic cerebral autoregulation associates with infarct size and outcome after ischemic stroke. *Acta Neurol Scand.* 2012;125(3):156–162.
3. Hlatky R, Valadka AB, Robertson CS. Intracranial pressure response to induced hypertension: role of dynamic pressure autoregulation. *Neurosurgery.* 2005;57(5):917–923.
4. Sviri GE, Newell DW. Cerebral autoregulation following traumatic brain injury. *The Open Neurosurgery Journal.* 2010;3:6–9.
5. Kalanuria A, Nyquist PA, Armonda RA, et al. Use of Transcranial Doppler (TCD) Ultrasound in the Neurocritical Care Unit. *Neurosurg Clin N Am.* 2013;24(3):441–456.
6. Purkayastha S, Sorond F. Transcranial Doppler ultrasound: technique and application. *Semin Neurol.* 2012;32(4):411–420.
7. Willie CK, Colino FL, Bailey DM, et al. Utility of transcranial Doppler ultrasound for the integrative assessment of cerebrovascular function. *J Neurosci Methods.* 2011;30, 196(2):221–237.
8. Matta BF, Lam AM, Strebel S, et al. Cerebral pressure autoregulation and carbon dioxide reactivity during propofol-induced EEG suppression. *Br J Anaesth.* 1995;74(2):159–163.
9. Sahuquillo J, Amoros S, Santos A, et al. False autoregulation (pseudoautoregulation) in patients with severe head injury. Its importance in CPP management. *Acta Neurochir Suppl.* 2000;76:485–490.
10. Puppo C, Fariña G, López FL, et al. Cerebral CO_2 reactivity in severe head injury. A transcranial Doppler study. *Acta Neurochir Suppl.* 2008;102:171–175.
11. Lee JH, Kelly DF, Oertel M, et al. Carbon dioxide reactivity, pressure autoregulation, and metabolic suppression reactivity after head injury: a transcranial Doppler study. *J Neurosurg.* 2001;95(2):222–232.
12. Czosnyka M, Brady K, Reinhard M, et al. Neurocrit Monitoring of cerebrovascular autoregulation: facts, myths, and missing links. Neurocrit Care. 2009;10(3):373–386.
13. Poon WS, Ng SC, Chan MT, et al. Cerebral blood flow (CBF)-directed management of ventilated head-injured patients. *Acta Neurochir Suppl.* 2005;95:9–11.

14. Asgari S, Bergsneider M, Hamilton R, et al. Consistent changes in intracranial pressure waveform morphology induced by acute hypercapnic cerebral vasodilatation. *Neurocrit Care*. 2011;15(1): 55–62.

15. Yoshihara M, Bandoh K, Marmarou A. Cerebrovascular carbon dioxide reactivity assessed by intracranial pressure dynamics in severely head injured patients. *J Neurosurg*. 1995;82(3):386–393.

16. Haubrich C, Steiner L, Kim DJ, et al. How does moderate hypocapnia affect cerebral autoregulation in response to changes in perfusion pressure in TBI patients? *Acta Neurochir Suppl*. 2012;114: 153–156.

17. Cho S, Fujigaki T, Uchiyama Y, et al. Effects of sevoflurane with and without nitrous oxide on human cerebral circulation. Transcranial Doppler study. *Anesthesiology*. 1996;85(4):755–760.

18. Aaslid R, Lindegaard KF, Sorteberg W, et al. Cerebral autoregulation dynamics in humans. *Stroke*. 1989;20(1):45–52.

19. Tiecks FP, Lam AM, Aaslid R, et al. Comparison of static and dynamic cerebral autoregulation measurements. *Stroke*. 1995;26(6):1014–1019.

20. Fraser CD 3rd, Brady KM, Rhee CJ, et al. The frequency response of cerebral autoregulation. *J Appl Physiol*. 2013;115(1):52–56.

21. Lewis PM, Smielewski P, Rosenfeld JV, et al. Monitoring of the association between cerebral blood flow velocity and intracranial pressure. *Acta Neurochir Suppl*. 2012;114:147–151.

22. Aries MJ, Czosnyka M, Budohoski KP, et al. Continuous monitoring of cerebrovascular reactivity using pulse waveform of intracranial pressure. *Neurocrit Care*. 2012;17(1):67–76.

23. Giller CA. A bedside test for cerebral autoregulation using transcranial Doppler ultrasound. *Acta Neurochir (Wien)*. 1991;108:7–14.

24. Czosnyka M, Pickard J, Whitehouse H, et al. The hyperaemic response to a transient reduction in cerebral perfusion pressure: a modelling study. *Acta Neurochir*. 1992;115:90–97.

25. Smielewski P, Czosnyka M, Kirkpatrick P, et al. Assessment of cerebral autoregulation using carotid artery compression. *Stroke*. 1996;27:2197–2203.

26. Smielewski P, Czosnyka M, Kirkpatrick P, et al. Evaluation of the transient hyperemic response test in head-injured patients. *J Neurosurg*. 1997;86(5):773–778.

27. Lam JM, Smielewski P, Czosnyka M, et al. Predicting delayed ischemic deficits after aneurysmal subarachnoid hemorrhage using a transient hyperemicresponse test of cerebral autoregulation. *Neurosurgery*. 2000;47(4):819–825.

28. Rasulo FA, Balestreri M, Matta B. Assessment of cerebral pressure autoregulation. *Curr Opin Anaesthesiol*. 2002;15(5):483–488.

29. Bouma GJ, Muizelaar JP, Bandoh K, et al: Blood pressure and intracranial pressure-volume dynamics in severe head injury: relationship with cerebral blood flow. *J Neurosurg*. 1992;77:15–19.

30. Reinhard M, Wehrle-Wieland E, Grabiak D, et al. Oscillatory cerebral hemodynamics—the macro- vs. microvascular level. *J Neurol Sci*. 2006;250(1–2):103–109.

31. Diehl RR, Linden D, Lucke D, et al. Phase relationship between cerebral blood flow velocity and blood pressure. A clinical test of autoregulation. *Stroke*. 1995;26(10):1801–1804.

32. Diehl RR, Linden D, Lucke D, et al. Spontaneous blood pressure oscillations and cerebral autoregulation. *Clin Auton Res*. 1998;8(1):7–12.

33. Kuo TB, Chern CM, Yang CC, et al. Mechanisms underlying phase lag between systemic arterial blood pressure and cerebral blood flow velocity. *Cerebrovasc Dis*. 2003;16(4):402–409.

34. Reinhard M, Roth M, Muller T, et al. Cerebral autoregulation in carotid artery occlusive disease assessed from spontaneous blood pressure fluctuations by the correlation coefficient index. *Stroke*. 2003;34(9):2138–2144.

35. Fàbregas N, Valero R, Carrero E, et al. Episodic high irrigation pressure during surgical neuroendoscopy may cause intermittent intracranial circulatory insufficiency. *J Neurosurg Anesthesiol*. 2001;13(2):152–157.

36. Fàbregas N, López A, Valero R, et al. Anesthetic management of surgical neuroendoscopies: usefulness of monitoring the pressure inside the neuroendoscope. *J Neurosurg Anesthesiol*. 2000;12(1): 21–28.

37. Salvador L, Hurtado P, Valero R, et al. Importance of monitoring neuroendoscopic intracranial pressure during anesthesia for neuroendoscopic surgery: review of 101 cases. *Rev Esp Anestesiol Reanim*. 2009;56(2):75–82.

38. Czosnyka M, Smielewski P, Kirkpatrick P, et al. Monitoring of cerebral autoregulation in head-injured patients. *Stroke.* 1996;27(10):1829–1834.
39. Czosnyka M, Smielewski P, Piechnik S, et al. Cerebral autoregulation following head injury. *J Neurosurg.* 2001;95(5):756–763.
40. Sviri GE, Aaslid R, Douville CM, et al. Time course for autoregulation recovery following severe traumatic brain injury. *J Neurosurg.* 2009;111:695–700.
41. Panerai RB, Kerins V, Fan L, et al. Association between dynamic cerebral autoregulation and mortality in severe head injury. *Br J Neurosurg.* 2004;18:471–479.
42. Steiger HJ, Aaslid R, Stooss R, et al. Transcranial Doppler monitoring in head injury: relations between type of injury, flow velocities, vasoreactivity, and outcome. *Neurosurgery.* 1994;34:79–85.
43. Czosnyka M, Smielewski P, Kirkpatrick P, et al. Continuous assessment of the cerebral vasomotor reactivity in head injury. *Neurosurgery.* 1997;41(1):11–17.
44. Lewis PM, Rosenfeld JV, Diehl RR, et al. Phase shift and correlation coefficient measurement of cerebral autoregulation during deep breathing in traumatic brain injury (TBI). *Acta Neurochir (Wien).* 2008;150(2):139–146.
45. Steiner LA, Coles JP, Johnston AJ, et al. Assessment of cerebrovascular autoregulation in head-injured patients: a validation study. *Stroke.* 2003;34(10):2404–2409.
46. Steiner LA, Coles JP, Czosnyka M, et al. Cerebrovascular pressure reactivity is related to global cerebral oxygen metabolism after head injury. *J Neurol Neurosurg Psychiatry.* 2003;74(6):765–770.
47. Timofeev I, Czosnyka M, Carpenter KL, et al. Interaction between brain chemistry and physiology after traumatic brain injury: impact of autoregulation and microdialysis catheter location. *J Neurotrauma.* 2011;28(6):849–860.
48. Piechnik S, Czosnyka M, Smielewski P, et al. Indices for decreased cerebral blood flow control—a modelling study. *Acta Neurochir Suppl.* 1998;71:269–271.
49. Steiner LA, Czosnyka M, Piechnik SK, et al. Continuous monitoring of cerebrovascular pressure reactivity allows determination of optimal cerebral perfusion pressure in patients with traumatic brain injury.*Crit Care Med.* 2002;30(4):733–738.
50. Overgaard J, Tweed WA. Cerebral circulation after head injury. 1. Cerebral blood flow and its regulation after closed head injury with emphasis on clinical correlations. *J Neurosurg.* 1974;41(5):531–541.
51. Aries MJ, Czosnyka M, Budohoski KP, et al. Continuous determination of optimal cerebral perfusion pressure in traumatic brain injury. *Crit Care Med.* 2012;40(8):2456–2463.
52. Brady KM, Shaffner DH, Lee JK, et al. Continuous monitoring of cerebrovascular pressure reactivity after traumatic brain injury in children. *Pediatrics.* 2009;124(6):e1205–e1212.
53. Oshorov AV, Savin IA, Goriachev AS, et al. The first experience in monitoring the cerebral vascular autoregulation in the acute period of severe brain injury. *Anesteziol Reanimatol.* 2008;(2):61–64.
54. Rao GS, Durga .P Changing trends in monitoring brain ischemia: from intracranial pressure to cerebral oximetry. *Curr Opin Anaesthesiol.* 2011;24(5):487–494.
55. Rosenthal G, Hemphill JC 3rd, Sorani M, et al. Brain tissue oxygen tension is more indicative of oxygen diffusion than oxygen delivery and metabolism in patients with traumatic brain injury. *Crit Care Med.* 2008;36(6):1917–1924.
56. Verweij BH, Amelink GJ, Muizelaar JP. Current concepts of cerebral oxygen transport and energy metabolism after severe traumatic brain injury. *Prog Brain Res.* 2007;161:111–124.
57. Yaseen MA, Srinivasan VJ, Sakadžić S, et al. Microvascular oxygen tension and flow measurements in rodent cerebral cortex during baselineconditions and functional activation. *J Cereb Blood Flow Metab.* 2011;31(4):1051–1063.
58. Haitsma IK, Maas AI: Monitoring cerebral oxygenation in traumatic brain injury. *Prog Brain Res.* 2007;161:207–216.
59. Hlatky R, Valadka AB, Gopinath SP, et al. Brain tissue oxygen tension response to induced hyperoxia reduced in hypoperfused brain. *J Neurosurg.* 2008;108:53–58.
60. van den Brink WA, van Santbrink H, Steyerberg EW, et al. Brain oxygen tension in severe head injury. *Neurosurgery.* 2000;46:868–876.
61. Stiefel MF, Spiotta A, Gracias VH, et al.Reduced mortality rate in patients with severe traumatic brain injury treated with brain tissue oxygen monitoring. *J Neurosurg.* 2005;103(5):805–811.

62. Narotam PK, Morrison JF, Nathoo N. Brain tissue oxygen monitoring in traumatic brain injury and major trauma: outcome analysis of a brain tissue oxygen-directed therapy. *J Neurosurg.* 2009;111(4): 672–682.

63. Lang EW, Czosnyka M, Mehdorn HM. Tissue oxygen reactivity and cerebral autoregulation after severe traumatic brain injury. *Crit Care Med.* 2003;31(1):267–271.

64. Jaeger M, Schuhmann MU, Soehle M, et al. Continuous assessment of cerebrovascular autoregulation after traumatic brain injury using brain tissue oxygen pressure reactivity. *J Crit Care Med.* 2006;34(6):1783–1788.

65. Radolovich DK, Czosnyka M, Timofeev I, et al. Reactivity of brain tissue oxygen to change in cerebral perfusion pressure in head injured patients. *Neurocrit Care.* 2009;10(3):274–279.

66. Jaeger M, Schuhmann MU, Soehle M, et al. Continuous monitoring of cerebrovascular autoregulation after subarachnoid hemorrhage by brain tissue oxygen pressure reactivity and its relation to delayed cerebral infarction. *Stroke.* 2007;38(3):981–986.

67. Jaeger M, Soehle M, Schuhmann MU, et al. Clinical significance of impaired cerebrovascular autoregulation after severe aneurysmal subarachnoid hemorrhage. *Stroke.* 2012; 43(8):2097–2101.

68. Ghosh A, Elwell C, Smith M. Review article: cerebral near-infrared spectroscopy in adults: a work in progress. *Anesth Analg.* 2012;115(6):1373–1383.

69. Murkin JM, Arango M Near-infrared spectroscopy as an index of brain and tissue oxygenation. *Br J Anaesth.* 2009; 103 Suppl 1:i3–i13.

70. Brady KM, Mytar JO, Kibler KK, et al. Noninvasive autoregulation monitoring with and without intracranial pressure in the naive piglet brain. *Anesth Analg.* 2010;111(1):191–195.

71. Steiner LA, Pfister D, Strebel SP, et al. Near-infrared spectroscopy can monitor dynamic cerebral autoregulation in adults. *Neurocrit Care.* 2009;10:122–128.

72. Joshi B, Ono M, Brown C, et al. Predicting the limits of cerebral autoregulation during cardiopulmonary bypass. *Anesth Analg.* 2012;114(3):503–510.

73. Brady K, Joshi B, Zweifel C, et al. Real-time continuous monitoring of cerebral blood flow autoregulation using near-infrared spectroscopy in patients undergoing cardiopulmonary bypass. *Stroke.* 2010;41(9):1951–1956.

74. Ono M, Arnaoutakis GJ, Fine DM, et al. Blood pressure excursions below the cerebral autoregulation threshold during cardiac surgery are associated with acute kidney injury. *Crit Care Med.* 2013;41(2):464–471.

75. Brady KM, Mytar JO, Lee JK, et al. Monitoring cerebral blood flow pressure autoregulation in pediatric patients during cardiac surgery. *Stroke.* 2010;41(9):1957–1962.

76. Lee JK, Kibler KK, Benni PB, et al. Cerebrovascular reactivity measured by near-infrared spectroscopy *Stroke.* 2009;40(5):1820–1826.

77. Diedler J, Zweifel C, Budohoski KP, et al. The limitations of near-infrared spectroscopy to assess cerebrovascular reactivity: the role of slow frequency oscillations. *Anesth Analg.* 2011;113(4): 849–857.

78. Zweifel C, Castellani G, Czosnyka M, et al. Noninvasive monitoring of cerebrovascular reactivity with near infrared spectroscopy in head-injured patients. *J Neurotrauma.* 2010;27(11):1951–1958.

79. Zweifel C, Castellani G, Czosnyka M, et al. Continuous assessment of cerebral autoregulation with near-infrared spectroscopy in adults after subarachnoid hemorrhage. *Stroke.* 2010;41(9):1963–1968.

80. Rhee CJ, Kibler KK, Brady KM, et al. Detection of neurologic injury using vascular reactivity monitoring and glial fibrillary acidicprotein. *Pediatrics.* 2013;131(3):e950–e954.

Neuroimaging

Latisha K. Ali, MD
David S. Liebeskind, MD

INTRODUCTION

In the management of neurological disorders, significant emphasis is placed on the importance of the clinical examination to identify the localization of a central or peripheral lesion. This is a critical step in acute neurologic disorders in guiding clinicians for emergent medical or surgical interventions. In critically ill patients, this is a challenging endeavor as many such individuals are sedated and/or paralyzed and the clinical exam may be difficult to ascertain.

Although relatively unexplored to date, monitoring of infarct patterns, hemorrhage evolution, and hemodynamics with serial imaging may be important for optimizing patient outcomes in the intensive care unit (ICU). Neuroimaging techniques have the potential to transform the management of ICU patients. Multimodal computed tomography (CT) and magnetic resonance imaging (MRI) rapidly illustrate the vascular and parenchymal correlates in acute ischemic and hemorrhagic stroke (Figures 8.1 and 8.2). Increasing use of multimodal imaging in the ICU has expanded our current understanding of stroke pathophysiology and streamlined the care of critically ill patients from the hyperacute to chronic phases. Multimodal CT and MRI, incorporating vascular and penumbral imaging, is useful for selection of intravenous thrombolytic and/or endovascular therapy. In addition, it may be used to identify patients at risk of early stroke or neurologic worsening requiring ICU admission, to prognosticate outcome, and to identify how frequently patients need to be monitored.

Surveillance imaging may even be useful in the absence of any clinical suspicion in comatose patients or those with known neurological illness or severe brain injury. Imaging may identify recurrent strokes, hemorrhagic transformation, or hemorrhage extension or other neurological injury. The use of advanced imaging approaches for early diagnosis and treatment of acute ischemic stroke also facilitates implementation of early secondary prevention algorithms. The mechanism or underlying subtype of ischemic stroke may be ascertained from

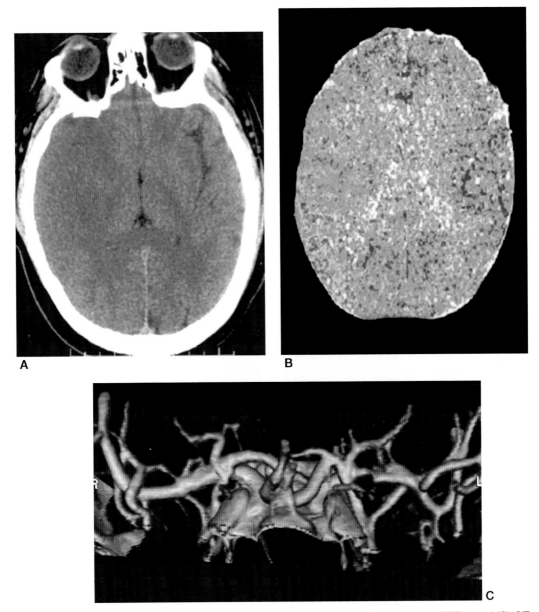

FIGURE 8.1 Multimodal CT, including (A) noncontrast CT, (B) CT perfusion (CTP), and (C) CT angiography (CTA), in acute stroke due to right middle cerebral artery distribution ischemia after partial reperfusion.

the use of multimodal imaging and allow for rapid implementation of secondary prevention measures. Imaging may also assist with prognostication and allow for planning of rehabilitation approaches as these advanced imaging modalities incorporate newer technologies that also provide information with regard to tissue metabolism and cerebrovascular reactivity.

ACUTE BRAIN INJURY ASSESSMENT

Imaging diagnosis of acute ischemic stroke complements the clinical examination by providing detailed information about the extent of evolving injury in the ischemic core and the potential therapeutic target of the surrounding penumbra or areas at risk. Both multimodal

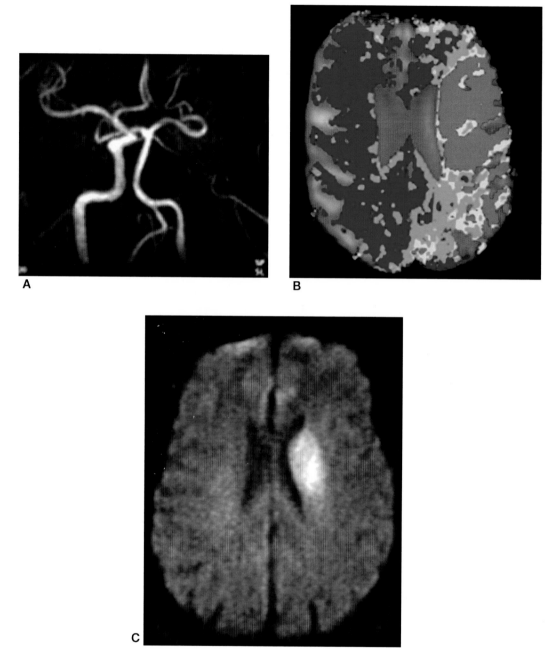

FIGURE 8.2 Multimodal MRI, including (A) time-of-flight MR angiography, (B) diffusion-weighted imaging, and (C) perfusion-weighted imaging (PWI), in acute stroke due to left middle cerebral artery occlusion.

CT and MRI can be used to confirm a diagnosis of stroke by documenting ischemic changes on noncontrast CT or diffusion-weighted imaging (DWI) sequences and can demonstrate the presence of arterial occlusion on angiography (Figures 8.3 and 8.4). One may also be able to estimate the degree of reduced blood flow with CT perfusion (CTP) or perfusion-weighted imaging (PWI).

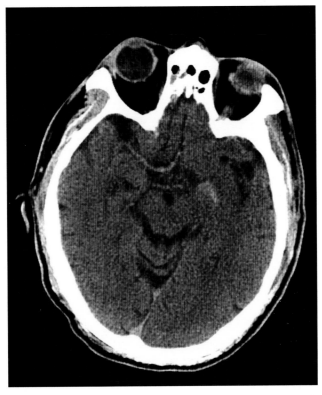

FIGURE 8.3 Dense right middle cerebral artery sign representing occlusion on noncontrast CT.

Noncontrast CT may be useful in detecting subtle signs of arterial occlusion and acute ischemia, including obscuration of the lentiform nuclei, hypoattenuation of the insular ribbon, sulcal effacement, cortical hypodensity, and various hyperdense vessel signs (1–4). Importantly, rapid diagnostic evaluation with CT reliably serves to rule out intracranial hemorrhage. Ischemic brain tissue is evident as hypodensity on noncontrast CT due to the influx of water associated with cerebral edema. Such changes typically manifest at about 6 hours after stroke onset. MRI sequences provide additional information on tissue characterization. DWI can demonstrate ischemic changes within minutes of stroke onset (5–8). Although DWI also has specificity for ischemia in excess of 90%, migraine, seizures, and other disease processes can be associated with DWI hyperintense lesions. The diagnosis of ischemia may be confirmed by finding corresponding hypointense lesions in a vascular distribution on apparent diffusion coefficient (ADC) maps.

VESSEL IMAGING

CT or MR Angiography

Multimodal CT, including CT angiography (CTA) and CTP, can be used to demonstrate the cerebrovascular anatomy in exquisite detail. CTA employs a timed bolus of iodinated contrast material to opacify vascular structures. Source images or raw axial data of enhanced

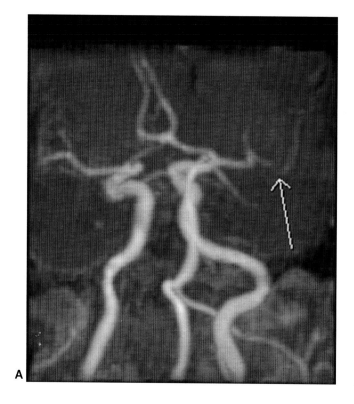

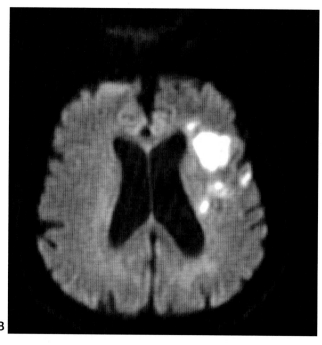

FIGURE 8.4 Left middle cerebral artery occlusion on MR angiography (A) with subsequent infarction demonstrated on DWI sequence (B).

vascular structures and postprocessed two-and three-dimensional reconstructions permit rapid identification of proximal occlusion (9–11). Early vessel signs, including the hyperdense MCA (middle cerebral artery) sign on a CT or a blooming artifact on gradient echo (GRE) MRI, may indicate red cell–rich thrombotic occlusions rather than fibrin-laden blockages (12). Practical approaches include consideration of clinical CT and clinical DWI mismatches in which the severity of the neurologic deficit is compared with the extent and location of the lesion on imaging (13–15). Severe deficits with small lesions strongly suggest a large area of hypoperfusion that affects potentially reversible tissues.

PERFUSION IMAGING

CTP utilizes iodinated material to track the influx of contrast-labeled arterial blood in the brain. Acquisition of serial images permits the generation of time-intensity curves for contrast passage through the brain. An arterial input function is selected for deconvolution and subsequent generation of perfusion parameters for each voxel. Perfusion maps are then constructed and various hemodynamic perfusion parameters, including mean transit time, cerebral blood volume, and cerebral blood flow are derived. Multimodal CT not only detects the absence of hemorrhage and the presence of ischemia, but also provides information on vascular anatomy and perfusion deficits.

Perfusion imaging with either CTP or PWI identify indirect markers of salvageable tissue constructed from mismatch combinations between clinical findings and CT, DWI, and vessel occlusion on MR angiography to suggest the presence of hypoperfusion in the affected territory. Arterial spin-labeled (ASL) perfusion imaging uses endogenous labeling of blood flow in the proximal arteries to measure downstream perfusion without the need for exogenous contrast agent (16,17). This technique can be easily repeated to measure changes in blood flow (Figure 8.5).

All perfusion imaging techniques may be limited by poor contrast opacification or timing errors due to decreased cardiac output, curtailed acquisitions that fail to capture the influential venous stages of perfusion, patient motion, and permeability changes in the blood–brain barrier (BBB). Perhaps the most significant limitation in perfusion imaging with either CT or MRI is the variability of results produced by different postprocessing software packages.

HYPERPERFUSION

Perfusion imaging may be useful in identifying patients with hyperperfusion who may be at risk of hemorrhagic transformation (18). After thrombolysis or other revascularization therapies, patients may be evaluated with repeated imaging during their ICU course. Monitoring the response to various acute stroke therapies may be facilitated with the use of multimodal CT/MRI. Serial imaging is helpful to characterize the dynamic nature if ischemia. Clinical response can be difficult to predict. Patients may have resolution of symptoms or rapid improvement due to arterial recanalization, but some may improve with head down-positioning, owing to improved residual flow or collateral perfusion despite persisting proximal arterial occlusion (Figure 8.6). There are many causes of early neurologic deterioration that may be disclosed with serial imaging. Infarct growth or hemorrhage

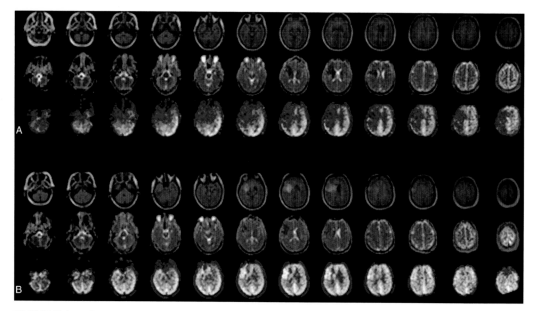

FIGURE 8.5 Serial MRI at (A) baseline and (B) 3 hours after revascularization of right-middle cerebral artery distribution stroke, revealing FLAIR evolution of ischemia (top rows) with ADC evidence of ischemic injury (middle rows) and ASL perfusion evidence (bottom rows) of hypoperfusion changing to hyperperfusion after treatment.

may be measured with serial or repeated parenchymal imaging, recanalization may be observed with serial noninvasive angiography imaging, and reperfusion may be identified with repeat CTP or PWI.

ASSESSMENT OF INTRACEREBRAL HEMORRHAGE

Multimodal CT and MRI may also be useful in hemorrhagic stroke assessment. Hematoma volume may be approximated by measuring the largest length and width on a single imaging slice, multiplying each by the vertical span of the clot, and dividing by two. Alternatively, volumetric software exists that provides more precise quantification of hematoma volumes. The CTA spot sign may predict hematoma expansion and perihematomal changes on CT/MRI of edema expansion (19,20). GRE MRI sequences may detect hemorrhage due to the susceptibility effects of blood products. GRE sequences may be equivalent to CT for detection and characterization of intracerebral hemorrhage (21–25). MRI can also provide information as to the cause of the spontaneous parenchymal hemorrhage such as vascular lesions or tumors. The presence and pattern of prior asymptomatic hemorrhages on GRE may be helpful in establishing the diagnosis of hypertensive (Figure 8.7) or cerebral amyloid angiopathy (CAA)-related hemorrhage (Figure 8.8).

The use of multimodal imaging in acute stroke has also influenced the clinical management of patients into subsequent phases. Acute therapy is primarily aimed at reversing the vascular occlusion with thrombolysis and/or thrombectomy. In intracerebral hemorrhage, antihypertensive measures are initiated to limit potential hematoma expansion.

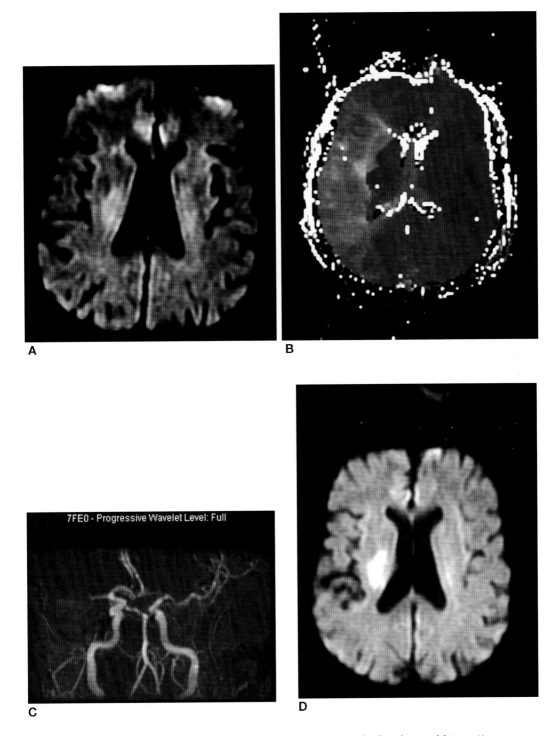

FIGURE 8.6 DWI (A) demonstrated recent ischemic change in the deep white matter. The PWI (B) showed mismatch in the entire right middle cerebral artery territory. The MR angiography (C) revealed abrupt occlusion of the right M1 segment. The patient had rapid improvement in clinical examination, possibly related to head-down positioning. She was treated with supportive care and (D) 3-hour follow-up MRI revealed no new lesions and improvement in the DWI abnormality.

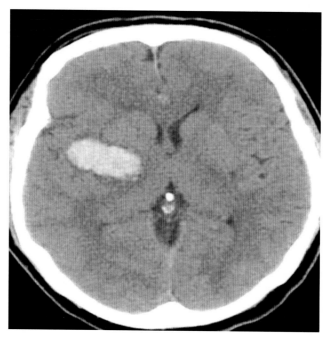

FIGURE 8.7 Noncontrast head CT of right putaminal spontaneous intraparenchymal hemorrhage.

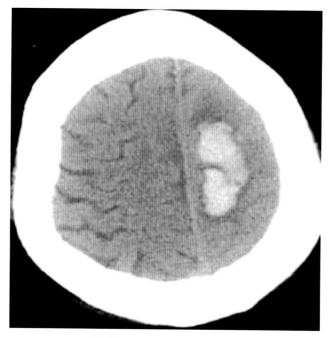

FIGURE 8.8 Noncontrast head CT of a cortically based, right hemispheric hemorrhage due to cerebral amyloid angiopathy.

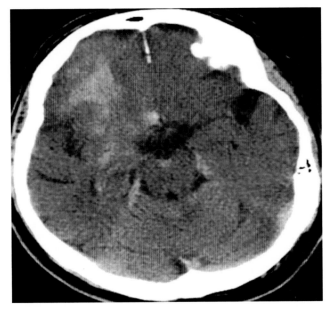

FIGURE 8.9 Noncontrast head CT of hemorrhagic transformation of a right frontal infarction follow interventional revascularization.

Hemodynamic interventions in subacute stroke are frequently determined based on imaging. Secondary complications are frequently discovered via imaging during the subacute phase (Figure 8.9). For instance, hemorrhagic transformation is commonly depicted with follow-up studies. This information is useful to guide secondary therapeutic decisions such as timing of antihypertensive and antithrombotic management. Considerations for subacute and subsequent management are therefore largely determined by the results of early imaging studies.

SERIAL IMAGING

Serial imaging of intracerebral hemorrhage is typically dictated by changes in the clinical examination. Follow-up CT scans are commonly ordered for patients in the neurointensive care unit when there is any concern for hematoma expansion or mass effect (Figure 8.10). Occasionally, such patients require subacute surgical interventions. Surgical decompression may be performed in the subacute period for mass effect due to cerebellar hemorrhage. Follow-up imaging may also be utilized to uncover or rule out the possibility of an underlying vascular lesion. In situations such as lobar hemorrhage in a younger patient, follow-up imaging may be necessary to reveal an underlying vascular lesion initially obscured by surrounding hemorrhage.

Antithrombotic management following intracerebral hemorrhage may also be influenced by imaging acquired during the subacute period. Although antithrombotic agents are generally withheld in the early stages after a hemorrhagic stroke, many such cases eventually require such therapy. Following a hypertensive hemorrhage, an individual may be at

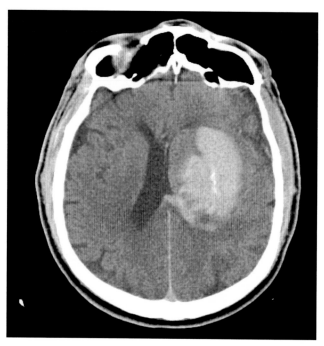

FIGURE 8.10 CT spot sign after spontaneous left basal ganglia intracerebral hemorrhage.

further risk of subsequent ischemic events. Imaging during the acute phase may uncover coexistent small-vessel ischemic disease or large-vessel atherosclerosis that requires antithrombotic therapy. Prior to the advent of multimodal imaging, most hemorrhage cases were evaluated with noncontrast CT, which provides only a limited extent of information regarding ischemia-related pathology. The addition of either CTA or MRI/MR angiography may provide a much greater extent of information regarding overall stroke risk.

Although most of the research and recent developments in stroke neuroimaging have focused on the hyperacute or acute stages, such technological advances have also substantially altered stroke care in the subacute phase and beyond. The early subacute time period is a dynamic phase during which many of the pathophysiological changes due to ischemia and acute treatments continue and offer an opportunity for intervention. Serial imaging may demonstrate progression of ischemia, recurrent stroke in previously unaffected territories, or, rarely, regression of initial lesions as in the case of DWI reversal associated with successful thrombolysis or spontaneous recanalization. Adverse effects of acute therapy may also be demonstrated during this period. Hemorrhagic transformation of an ischemic infarct may result from thrombolytic therapy.

During the early subacute period, cytotoxic and vasogenic edema evolve within the ischemic zone. Progressive edema may exacerbate injury in adjacent regions and occasionally lead to herniation. Although several interventions for edema following ischemic stroke are utilized, such as mannitol, hyperventilation, or hemicraniectomy, there are no established neuroimaging criteria to guide management.

Hemorrhagic transformation due to extensive ischemia and reperfusion or thrombolytic therapy may occur during the subacute phase. Noncontrast CT is routinely acquired 24 hours after administration of intravenous tPA for surveillance of hemorrhagic transformation. It is important to obtain an imaging study such as CT or GRE 24 hours after any intervention as evidence of hemorrhage may affect antithrombotic decisions. At some centers, in addition to the 24-hour CT, a follow-up scan employing multimodal CT or MRI may be obtained several days after an acute intervention. This invaluable information may promote the use of early serial scanning as part of clinical routine. Such scans have shown that, in a minority of patients, recanalized vessels may reocclude and occluded vessels may spontaneously recanalize. This information may substantially impact subsequent long-term care. For instance, a patient on anticoagulation therapy for a carotid dissection may no longer need to be on anticoagulation if the vessel is noted to be completely occluded on follow-up imaging. Conversely, an occluded carotid due to atherosclerotic disease may subsequently recanalize, prompting treatment of an underlying plaque.

The initial imaging during the acute phase may rapidly identify an underlying cause of transient ischemic attack (TIA) or stroke etiology. Imaging studies utilizing ultrasonography, CT, MRI, or angiography provide not only information about stroke etiology, but also overall ischemic and hemorrhagic stroke risk. Various modalities may reveal carotid stenosis that may be treated with subacute intervention, including either carotid endarterectomy or stenting. Early detection of scattered microhemorrhages on GRE may suggest prominent hypertensive disease or CAA (cerebral amyloid angiopathy). Deeply situated microhemorrhages may suggest hypertensive sequelae, whereas lobar or more diffuse lesions may suggest CAA. The presence of scattered microbleeds on GRE associated with CAA may preclude anticoagulation due to the risk of hemorrhage.

TRAUMATIC BRAIN INJURY

Traumatic brain injury (TBI) is a major cause of death and permanent disability worldwide. It has been referred to as the "silent epidemic" as it is often not recognized and is underreported.

The Centers for Disease Control and Prevention (CDC) estimates it occurs in 1.7 million people annually in the United States and accrues medical costs in excess of $60 billion each year (26–28).

Imaging is useful not only to identify the acute injury to the brain but also as surveillance imaging to identify secondary injuries such as cerebral herniation, cerebral edema, hydrocephalus, and hemorrhage, and to serially monitor any progression. Imaging also guides rehabilitation therapies and determines prognosis and management of sequelae in chronic TBI patients (29).

Neuroimaging may not be required in all patients with head trauma but there is often debate in defining these patients. Determining the specific patients who may benefit is essential (30–33) as Nagy (34) and others have reported that less than 10% of patients with minor head injuries have positive findings on CT and less than 1% will require neurosurgical interventions (34,35). Differentiating and defining major and minor head trauma can be difficult. There are many criteria, including the Canadian Head CT rules and the New Orleans criteria (36–44) to help with such differentiation. If a patient has a low score on the

Glasgow Coma Scale (45) clinical characteristics such as the loss or altered level of consciousness, amnesia, focal neurologic findings, emesis, headache, seizures, skull injuries or fractures, ethanol or drug intoxication, age > 60 years or in infants, then neuroimaging is generally recommended (35,36,46–56).

In most acute cases, CT is the initial modality utilized to identify intracranial hemorrhage (30,31,57,58). It is readily available and more cost effective, requires shorter imaging time, and is easier to acquire in ventilated or agitated patients (29). CT can easily differentiate extra-axial hemorrhage (epidural, subdural, subarachnoid and intraventricular hemorrhage) and intra-axial hemorrhage (intraparenchymal hematoma, contusions, and shear injury) (57). Limitations of CT include beam-hardening artifacts, distortion of signal near bone and metal, the potential to miss small amounts of blood, and the fact that findings may lag behind tissue damage or underestimate the degree of injury (29,59–61).

MRI is sensitive in diagnosing TBI and is considered superior to CT in the subacute and chronic management of these patients. MRI is useful in detecting brainstem lesions, axonal injury, contusions, and subtle neuronal damage (62,63). MRI has identified injury missed in 10% to 20% of CT (57,63–65).

Either hemorrhage or cerebral edema may cause mass effect, thereby compromising vascular structures culminating in ischemia and infarction or compressing structures leading to herniation. Imaging is important in assessing these patients as there is often progression or delayed compromise and repeat neuroimaging is warranted.

Cerebral contusions are scattered areas of bleeding on the surface of the brain, most commonly along the undersurface and poles of the frontal and temporal lobes. Contusions may occur in over 40% of patients with blunt trauma and as coup-contrecoup injuries in deceleration or acceleration trauma (66). On noncontrast CT (Figure 8.11), contusions

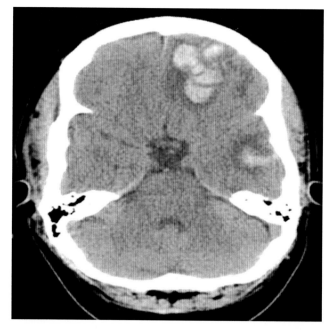

FIGURE 8.11 Noncontrast head CT of left frontal and temporal traumatic contusions.

appear as areas of low attenuation if hemorrhage is absent and mixed or high attenuation if hemorrhage is present. In the acute stage, CT is more sensitive than MRI, as the clot signal can be indistinguishable from brain parenchyma on MRI. After the first few hours, the hemoglobin in the contusion loses its oxygen to become deoxyhemoglobin, which is still not well visualized on T1-weighted MRI, but the concentration of red blood cells and fibrin can cause low signal on T2-weighted images. Over the next several days, as the contusion liquefies and the deoxyhemoglobin oxidizes to methemoglobin that is strongly paramagnetic, the contusion becomes more easily visualized on MRI (Figure 8.12; 29,67,68).

Subdural hematomas (Figure 8.13) occur in 10% to 20% of patients with head trauma and are associated with high mortality (69). In the subacute stage, subdural hematomas approach the attenuation of normal brain parenchyma and MRI becomes more effective than CT in detection (70).

Subarachnoid hemorrhage (SAH; Figure 8.14) refers to blood within the subarachnoid space from any pathologic process. The most common source of SAH is trauma. Traumatic SAH must be distinguished from rupture of a saccular aneurysm or arteriovenous malformation, as management of the latter differs considerably. Emergent control of the bleeding source is critical as 10% to 15% of patients die before reaching the hospital and mortality rates in the first week are as high as 40% (71–74). CT is superior to conventional MRI sequences in detecting acute SAH because the blood in acute SAH has a low hematocrit and low deoxyhemoglobin, which makes it appear similar to brain parenchyma on T1- and T2-weighted spin echo images. However, FLAIR (Figure 8.15) sequences may find small acute or subacute SAH missed by CT and conventional MRI (29,70,75,76).

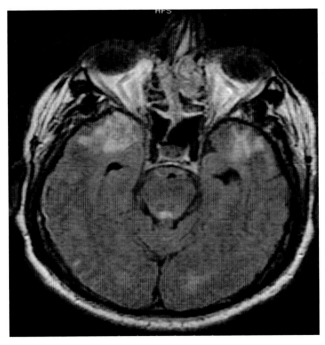

FIGURE 8.12 MRI FLAIR sequence image of subacute bilateral temporal contusions.

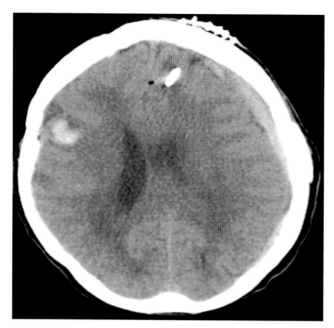

FIGURE 8.13 Noncontrast head CT demonstrating a left hemispheric acute subdural hemorrhage.

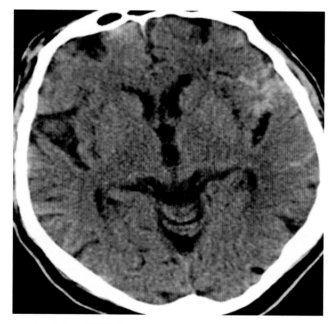

FIGURE 8.14 Noncontrast head CT demonstrating traumatic subarachnoid blood in the left sylvian fissure and overlying cortical surface.

Epidural hematomas (EDH; Figure 8.16) occur in 1% to 4% of patients and are not very common. It is generally recommended to conservatively manage patients who exhibit an EDH that is less than 30 mL, less than 15-mm thick, and less than 5-mm midline shift, without a focal neurologic deficit and GCS greater than 8 (75–79).

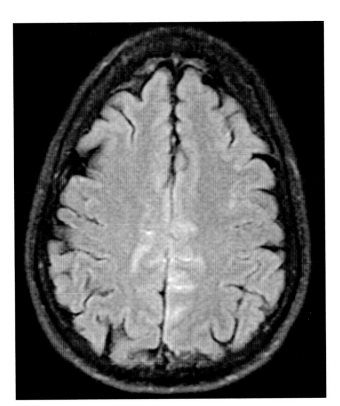

FIGURE 8.15 MRI FLAIR sequence image of midline traumatic subarachnoid blood.

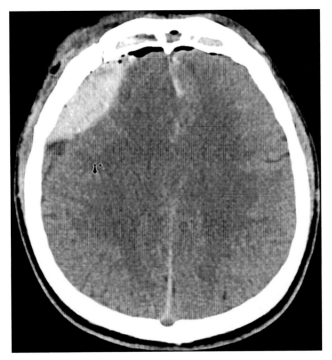

FIGURE 8.16 Noncontrast head CT of right frontal traumatic epidural hemorrhage with overlying nondisplaced skull fracture.

Fractures are important to identify and may need to be surgically repaired based on location, size, or type of fracture. Plain films of the skull may detect fractures but CT is recommended to assess for fracture. Fractures involving the paranasal sinuses, mastoid air cells, or the entire thickness of the calvarium can allow air to enter the intracranial space. Air appears as an area of low attenuation on CT and signal void on MRI. If persistent, cerebral sinus fluid leak is usually suspect. It is recommended that basilar skull fractures receive a follow-up CT scan to exclude pneumocephalus (80,81).

VASCULAR INJURY

Fistulae, dissections, or aneurysms may result from trauma. Contrast angiography has been the gold standard for diagnosis of vascular lesions but non invasive testing with MRI, MR angiography, and (CTA; Figure 8.17) are useful as well and provide additional information about the arterial walls and MRI about the adjoining brain parenchyma (82–84). Imaging is also useful to understand the anatomy and guide surgical approaches (29,85,86).

CHRONIC MANAGEMENT OF TRAUMTIC BRAIN INJURY

Imaging can guide chronic TBI management by identifying late complications such as chronic or delayed hemorrhage. It is useful in guiding rehabilitation and understanding prognosis and possibly functional outcome. Diffuse axonal injury (DAI) occurs in almost half of patients with closed head injuries. It is caused by the sheer force generated by the rapid deceleration in motor vehicle accidents (64). DAI can result in significant neurologic impairment and the number of lesions correlates with poorer outcomes. CT is useful to visualize hemorrhagic injury but MRI is more sensitive for detecting neuronal damage and diffusion tensor imaging may also be useful as well (87–90).

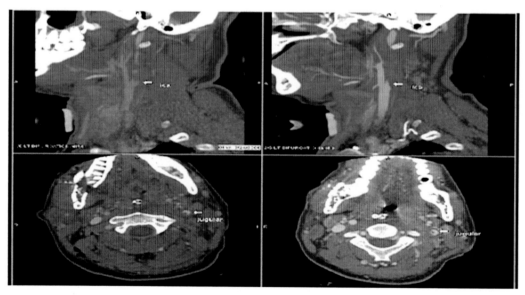

FIGURE 8.17 CTA images of left carotid occlusion distal to the bifurcation resulting from vascular dissection following a penetrating gunshot wound to the neck.

RESEARCH IMAGING MODALITIES

Diffusion Tensor Imaging

Diffusion tensor imaging (DTI) is a technique that uses six or more isotropic diffusion-weighted images to describe the microstructural integrity of axons within white matter. White matter tractography is a postprocessing technique applied to DTI that allows for the mathematical reconstruction of white matter tracts. DTI tractography applied to patients at an acute-to-subacute timepoint of less than 12 hours after symptom onset focused on pyramidal tract integrity found that disrupted white matter integrity correlated closely with motor function outcome (91,92). DTI remains a research imaging protocol, but this method is currently under investigation as a marker of potential functional outcome and as a marker of ischemia in acute ischemic stroke.

RESTING STATE FUNCTIONAL MRI

Resting state functional MRI may be used to assess tissue viability and potential for recovery. Golestani et al obtained resting state MRI for stroke patients acutely and after 90 days. In patients with motor symptoms, interhemispheric connectivity was impaired, and in patients with recovery of motor function, connectivity was reestablished (93). Resting state MRI remains a research protocol, but in the future this approach could predict ultimate outcomes or guide functional therapies.

PORTABLE NEUROIMAGING

Transportation of ICU patients for serial imaging is often associated with significant logistical and safety issues (94–97). Transportation may exacerbate pulmonary function, compromise intracranial physiology or aggravate outcome (96,97). Peace et al demonstrated that the use of a portable CT scan has little to no effect on intracranial pressure, cerebral perfusion pressure, or brain tissue oxygen pressure. As such, portable HCT (Figure 8.18) may be helpful in reducing the risk of secondary insult in the ICU patient (94,96,97).

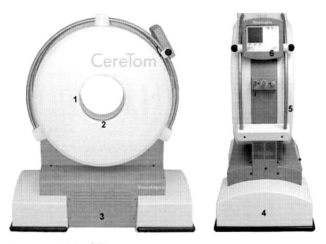

FIGURE 8.18 Ceretom portable CT scanner.

REFERENCES

1. Patel SC, et al. Lack of clinical significance of early ischemic changes on computed tomography in acute stroke. *JAMA*.2001;286(22):2830–2838.
2. Kalafut MA, et al. Detection of early CT signs of >1/3 middle cerebral artery infarctions: interrater reliability and sensitivity of CT interpretation by physicians involved in acute stroke care. *Stroke*. 2000;31(7):1667–1671.
3. Tomsick TA, et al. Hyperdense middle cerebral artery: incidence and quantitative significance. *Neuroradiology*. 1989;31(4):312–315.
4. von Kummer R, et al. Sensitivity and prognostic value of early CT in occlusion of the middle cerebral artery trunk. *AJNR Am J Neuroradiol*. 1994;15(1):9–15; discussion 16–18.
5. Warach S, et al. Time course of diffusion imaging abnormalities in human stroke. *Stroke*. 1996; 27(7):1254–1256.
6. Warach S, Dashe JF, and Edelman RR, Clinical outcome in ischemic stroke predicted by early diffusion-weighted and perfusion magnetic resonance imaging: a preliminary analysis. *J Cereb Blood Flow Metab*. 1996;16(1):53–59.
7. Warach S., Boska M, and Welch KM, Pitfalls and potential of clinical diffusion-weighted MR imaging in acute stroke. *Stroke*. 1997;28(3):481–482.
8. Baird AE, et al. Enlargement of human cerebral ischemic lesion volumes measured by diffusion-weighted magnetic resonance imaging. *Ann Neurol*. 1997;41(5):581–589.
9. Knauth M, et al. Potential of CT angiography in acute ischemic stroke. *AJNR Am J Neuroradiol*. 1997;18(6):1001–1010.
10. Verro P, et al. CT angiography in acute ischemic stroke: preliminary results. *Stroke*. 2002;33(1): 276–278.
11. Verro P, et al. Clinical application of CT angiography in acute ischemic stroke. *Clin Neurol Neurosurg*. 2007;109(2):138–145.
12. Liebeskind DS, et al. CT and MRI early vessel signs reflect clot composition in acute stroke. *Stroke*. 2011;42(5):1237–1243.
13. Choi JY, et al. Does clinical-CT 'mismatch' predict early response to treatment with recombinant tissue plasminogen activator? *Cerebrovasc Dis*. 2006;22(5–6):384–388.
14. Rodriguez-Yanez M, et al. Early biomarkers of clinical-diffusion mismatch in acute ischemic stroke. *Stroke*. 2011;42(10):2813–2818.
15. Davalos A, et al. The clinical-DWI mismatch: a new diagnostic approach to the brain tissue at risk of infarction. *Neurology*. 2004;62(12):2187–2192.
16. Zaharchuk G, et al. Arterial spin labeling imaging findings in transient ischemic attack patients: comparison with diffusion- and bolus perfusion-weighted imaging. *Cerebrovasc Dis*. 2012;34(3): 221–228.
17. Zaharchuk G. Arterial spin label imaging of acute ischemic stroke and transient ischemic attack. *Neuroimaging Clin N Am*. 2011;21(2):285–301, x.
18. Kidwell CS, et al. Diffusion-perfusion MRI characterization of post-recanalization hyperperfusion in humans. *Neurology*. 2001;57(11):2015–2021.
19. Demchuk AM, et al. Prediction of haematoma growth and outcome in patients with intracerebral haemorrhage using the CT-angiography spot sign (PREDICT): a prospective observational study. *Lancet Neurol*, 2012;11(4):307–314.
20. Chakraborty S, et al. Dynamic nature of the CT angiographic "spot sign". *Br J Radiol*. 2010;83(994): e216-219.
21. Kidwell CS, et al. Comparison of MRI and CT for detection of acute intracerebral hemorrhage. *JAMA*. 2004;292(15):1823–1830.
22. Fiebach JB., Steiner T, and Neumann-Haefelin T, [Neuroimaging evaluation of intracerebral hemorrhage]. *Nervenarzt*. 2009;80(2):205–213; quiz 214.
23. Fiebach JB et al. CT and diffusion-weighted MR imaging in randomized order: diffusion-weighted imaging results in higher accuracy and lower interrater variability in the diagnosis of hyperacute ischemic stroke. *Stroke*. 2002;33(9):2206–2210.
24. Fiebach JB, et al. Stroke magnetic resonance imaging is accurate in hyperacute intracerebral hemorrhage: a multicenter study on the validity of stroke imaging. *Stroke*. 2004;35(2):502–506.
25. Fiebach J, et al. Comparison of CT with diffusion-weighted MRI in patients with hyperacute stroke. *Neuroradiology*. 2001;43(8):628–632.

26. Centers for Disease Control and Prevention. CDC grand rounds: reducing severe traumatic brain injury in the United States. *MMWR Morb Mortal Wkly Rep.* 2013;62(27):549–552.

27. Coronado VG, et al. The CDC traumatic brain injury surveillance system: characteristics of persons aged 65 years and older hospitalized with a TBI. *J Head Trauma Rehabil.* 2005;20(3):215–228.

28. Langlois JA and Smith RW., Traumatic brain injury in the United States: research and programs of the Centers for Disease Control and Prevention (CDC). *J Head Trauma Rehabil.* 2005;20(3): 187-188.

29. Lee B and Newberg A. Neuroimaging in traumatic brain imaging. *NeuroRx.* 2005;2(2):372–383.

30. Miller EC, Derlet, RW, and Kinsert D. Minor head trauma: Is computed tomography always necessary? *Ann Emerg Med.* 1996;27(3):290–294.

31. Miller EC, Holmes JF, and Derlet RW. Utilizing clinical factors to reduce head CT scan ordering for minor head trauma patients. *J Emerg Med.* 1997;15(4):453–457.

32. Reinus WR, Erickson, KK, and Wippold FJ II. Unenhanced emergency cranial CT: optimizing patient selection with univariate and multivariate analyses. *Radiology.* 1993;186(3):763–768.

33. Reinus WR, et al. Emergency imaging of patients with resolved neurologic deficits: value of immediate cranial CT. *AJR Am J Roentgenol.* 1994;163(3):667–670.

34. Nagy KK, et al. The utility of head computed tomography after minimal head injury. *J Trauma.* 1999;46(2):268–270.

35. Jeret JS, et al. Clinical predictors of abnormality disclosed by computed tomography after mild head trauma. *Neurosurgery.* 1993;32(1):9–15; discussion 15–16.

36. Haydel MJ, et al. Indications for computed tomography in patients with minor head injury. *N Engl J Med.* 2000;343(2):100–105.

37. Stiell IG, et al. A prospective cluster-randomized trial to implement the Canadian CT Head Rule in emergency departments. *CMAJ.* 2010;182(14):1527–1532.

38. Stiell IG, et al. Comparison of the Canadian CT Head Rule and the New Orleans Criteria in patients with minor head injury. *JAMA.* 2005;294(12):1511–1518.

39. Stiell IG, et al. Indications for computed tomography after minor head injury. Canadian CT Head and Cervical-Spine Study Group. *N Engl J Med.* 2000;343(21):1570–1571.

40. Stiell IG, et al. Canadian CT head rule study for patients with minor head injury: methodology for phase II (validation and economic analysis). *Ann Emerg Med;* 2001;38(3):317–322.

41. Stiell IG, et al. The Canadian CT Head Rule Study for patients with minor head injury: rationale, objectives, and methodology for phase I (derivation). *Ann Emerg Med.* 2001;38(2):160–169.

42. Stiell IG, et al. The Canadian CT Head Rule for patients with minor head injury. *Lancet.* 2001; 357(9266):1391–1396.

43. De Kruijk JR., Twijnstra A, and Leffers P. Diagnostic criteria and differential diagnosis of mild traumatic brain injury. *Brain Inj.* 2001;15(2):99–106.

44. Mena JH, et al. Effect of the modified Glasgow Coma Scale score criteria for mild traumatic brain injury on mortality prediction: comparing classic and modified Glasgow Coma Scale score model scores of 13. *J Trauma.* 2011;71(5):1185–1192; discussion 1193.

45. Ingebrigtsen T, et al. Scandinavian guidelines for management of minimal, mild and moderate head injuries]. *Tidsskr Nor Laegeforen.* 2000;120(17):1985–1990.

46. Ingebrigtsen T, et al. Mild head injury. *J Neurosurg.* 2005;102(1):184; author reply 185.

47. Ingebrigtsen T and Romner B. Should brain injury markers replace CT in mild head injury?. *Tidsskr Nor Laegeforen.* 2012;132(17):1948–1949.

48. Ingebrigtsen T and Romner B. Routine early CT-scan is cost saving after minor head injury. *Acta Neurol Scand.* 1996;93(2–3):207–210.

49. Ingebrigtsen T, Romner B, and Trumpy JH. Management of minor head injury: the value of early computed tomography and serum protein S-100 measurements. *J Clin Neurosci.* 1997;4(1):29–33.

50. Schunk JE and Schutzman SA. Pediatric head injury. *Pediatr Rev.* 2012;33(9):398–410; quiz 410–411.

51. Moran SG, et al. Predictors of positive CT scans in the trauma patient with minor head injury. *Am Surg.* 1994;60(7):533–535; discussion 535–536.

52. Duus BR, et al. Prognostic signs in the evaluation of patients with minor head injury. *Br J Surg.* 1993; 80(8):988–991.

53. Duus BR, et al. The role of neuroimaging in the initial management of patients with minor head injury. *Ann Emerg Med.* 1994;23(6):1279–1283.

54. Haydel MJ. Clinical decision instruments for CT scanning in minor head injury. *JAMA*, 2005; 294(12):1551–1553.

55. Kraus JF, et al. Incidence, severity, and external causes of pediatric brain injury. *Am J Dis Child.* 1986;140(7):687–693.

56. Schonfeld D, et al. Pediatric Emergency Care Applied Research Network head injury clinical prediction rules are reliable in practice. *Arch Dis Child.* 2014;99(5):427–431.

57. Yealy DM and Hogan DE. Imaging after head trauma. Who needs what? *Emerg Med Clin North Am.* 1991;9(4):707–717.

58. Jones TR, et al. Single- versus multi-detector row CT of the brain: quality assessment. *Radiology.* 2001;219(3):750–755.

59. Lee H, et al. Focal lesions in acute mild traumatic brain injury and neurocognitive outcome: CT versus 3T MRI. *J Neurotrauma.* 2008;25(9):1049–1056.

60. Servadei F, et al. CT prognostic factors in acute subdural haematomas: the value of the 'worst' CT scan. *Br J Neurosurg.* 2000;14(2):110–116.

61. Figg RE, Burry, TS, and Vander Kolk WE.Clinical efficacy of serial computed tomographic scanning in severe closed head injury patients. *J Trauma.* 2003;55(6):1061–1064.

62. Levin HS, et al. Magnetic resonance imaging and computerized tomography in relation to the neurobehavioral sequelae of mild and moderate head injuries. *J Neurosurg.* 1987;66(5):706–713.

63. Ogawa T, et al. Comparative study of magnetic resonance and CT scan imaging in cases of severe head injury. *Acta Neurochir Suppl (Wien).* 1992;55:8–10.

64. Mittl RL, et al. Prevalence of MR evidence of diffuse axonal injury in patients with mild head injury and normal head CT findings. *AJNR Am J Neuroradiol.* 1994;15(8):1583–1589.

65. Doezema D, et al. Magnetic resonance imaging in minor head injury. *Ann Emerg Med.* 1991; 20(12):1281–1285.

66. Bruns J Jr and Hauser, WA. The epidemiology of traumatic brain injury: a review. *Epilepsia.* 2003; 44 Suppl 10, 2–10.

67. Bradley WG Jr. MR appearance of hemorrhage in the brain. *Radiology.* 1993;189(1):15–26.

68. Quencer RM and Bradley WG.MR imaging of the brain: what constitutes the minimum acceptable capability? *AJNR Am J Neuroradiol.* 2001;22(8):1449–1450.

69. Gutman MB, et al. Risk factors predicting operable intracranial hematomas in head injury. *J Neurosurg.* 1992;77(1):9–14.

70. Bakshi R, et al. Fluid-attenuated inversion-recovery MR imaging in acute and subacute cerebral intraventricular hemorrhage. *AJNR Am J Neuroradiol.* 1999;20(4):629–636.

71. Connolly ES Jr., et al. Guidelines for the management of aneurysmal subarachnoid hemorrhage: a guideline for healthcare professionals from the American Heart Association/American Stroke Association. *Stroke.* 2012;43(6):1711–17137.

72. Naval NS, et al. Improved aneurysmal subarachnoid hemorrhage outcomes: a comparison of 2 decades at an academic center. *J Crit Care.* 2013;28(2):182–188.

73. Naval NS, et al. Impact of pattern of admission on outcomes after aneurysmal subarachnoid hemorrhage. *J Crit Care.* 2012;27(5):e1–e7.

74. Naval NS, et al. Controversies in the management of aneurysmal subarachnoid hemorrhage. *Crit Care Med.* 2006;34(2):511–524.

75. Ashikaga R. [Clinical utility of MR FLAIR imaging for head injuries]. *Nihon Igaku Hoshasen Gakkai Zasshi.* 1996;56(14):1045–1049.

76. Ashikaga R, Araki Y, and Ishida O, MRI of head injury using FLAIR. *Neuroradiology.* 1997;39(4):239–242.

77. Bullock MR, et al. Surgical management of acute epidural hematomas. *Neurosurgery.* 2006; 58(3 Suppl):S7–15; discussion Si–Siv.

78. Offner PJ, Pham, B, and Hawkes A., Nonoperative management of acute epidural hematomas: a "no-brainer". *Am J Surg.* 2006; 92(6):801–805.

79. Chen TY, et al. The expectant treatment of "asymptomatic" supratentorial epidural hematomas. *Neurosurgery.* 1993;32(2):176–179; discussion 179.

80. Gruen P. Surgical management of head trauma. *Neuroimaging Clin N Am.* 2002;12(2):339–343.

81. Zee CS, et al. Imaging of sequelae of head trauma. *Neuroimaging Clin N Am.* 2002;12(2):325–338, ix.

82. Sa de Camargo EC and Koroshetz WJ, Neuroimaging of ischemia and infarction. *NeuroRx.* 2005; 2(2):265–276.

83. Biffl WL and Moore EE. Identifying the asymptomatic patient with blunt carotid arterial injury. *J Trauma*. 1999;47(6):1163–1164.

84. Rogers FB, et al. Computed tomographic angiography as a screening modality for blunt cervical arterial injuries: preliminary results. *J Trauma*. 1999;46(3):380–385.

85. Guyot LL, Kazmierczak CD, and Diaz FG. Vascular injury in neurotrauma. *Neurol Res*. 2001; 23(2–3):291–296.

86. Wellwood J, Alcantara A, and Michael DB, Neurotrauma: the role of CT angiogram. *Neurol Res*. 2002;24 Suppl 1:S13–S16.

87. Luccichenti G, et al. 3 Tesla is twice as sensitive as 1.5 Tesla magnetic resonance imaging in the assessment of diffuse axonal injury in traumatic brain injury patients. *Funct Neurol*. 2010;25(2): 109–114.

88. Topal NB, et al. MR imaging in the detection of diffuse axonal injury with mild traumatic brain injury. *Neurol Res*. 2008;30(9):974–978.

89. Inglese M, et al. Diffuse axonal injury in mild traumatic brain injury: a diffusion tensor imaging study. *J Neurosurg*. 2005;103(2):298–303.

90. McGowan JC, et al. Diffuse axonal pathology detected with magnetization transfer imaging following brain injury in the pig. *Magn Reson Med*. 1999;41(4):727–733.

91. Puig J, et al. Wallerian degeneration in the corticospinal tract evaluated by diffusion tensor imaging correlates with motor deficit 30 days after middle cerebral artery ischemic stroke. *AJNR Am J Neuroradiol*. 2010;31(7):1324–1330.

92. Puig J, et al. Acute damage to the posterior limb of the internal capsule on diffusion tensor tractography as an early imaging predictor of motor outcome after stroke. *AJNR Am J Neuroradiol*. 2011; 32(5):857–863.

93. Golestani AM, et al. Longitudinal evaluation of resting-state FMRI after acute stroke with hemiparesis. *Neurorehabil Neural Repair*. 2013;27(2):153–163.

94. Andrews PJ, et al. Secondary insults during intrahospital transport of head-injured patients. *Lancet*. 1990;335(8685):327–330.

95. Bercault N, et al. Intrahospital transport of critically ill ventilated patients: a risk factor for ventilator-associated pneumonia—a matched cohort study. *Crit Care Med*. 2005;33(11):2471–2478.

96. Peace K, et al. The use of a portable head CT scanner in the intensive care unit. J *Neurosci Nurs*. 2010;42(2):109–116.

97. Peace K, et al. Portable head CT scan and its effect on intracranial pressure, cerebral perfusion pressure, and brain oxygen. *J Neurosurg*. 2011;114(5):1479–1484.

Evoked Potentials in Neurocritical Care

Wei Xiong, MD
Matthew Eccher, MD, MSPH
Romergryko Geocadin, MD

INTRODUCTION

Evoked potentials (EP) are a reliable and informative method of evaluating and monitoring patients in a neurologic intensive care unit (ICU). EPs test the intactness of neurologic pathways in and out of a patient's brain. They range from the commonly used somatosensory evoked potentials (SSEP), which test the afferent peripheral sensory pathways, to motor evoked potentials (MEP), which test the efferent motor output conduits. Sensory EPs can also be generally divided into short and long latency, where the short-latency components represent the direct projection of sensory input into the subcortical structures and primary sensory cortices, and the long-latency components represent higher cognitive and cortical processing (1–3).

Compared to other electrophysiologic monitoring methods such as electroencephalography (EEG), EP are more resistant to sedatives and anesthetics (4–6). For a patient who is pharmacologically paralyzed and sedated, following the clinical exam—the gold-standard of monitoring in the neurologic ICU—would be impossible and, at best, unreliable. On the other hand, EPs have the advantage of being unaffected by (and even enhanced by) paralytic agents. EPs are not a replacement for a good neurologic examination, but when used prudently, can provide insight into pathways otherwise not assessable clinically. While EP monitoring is often helpful, its utility is limited to assessment of the specific system that it queries (eg, somatosensory system and its projection to the cortex).

EP signals are often low in amplitude and, therefore, suffer from low signal-to-noise ratios (SNR) without additional processing. The fact that they are time-locked to an artificial stimulus allows them to be averaged over hundreds of trials, dramatically boosting their SNR even in electronically noisy ICU environments (7). This quality is essential in today's multimodal-monitored ICU.

TYPES OF EVOKED POTENTIALS

Somatosensory Evoked Potentials (SSEP)

The most extensively used and studied EP in the neurologic ICU is the SSEP. Their ease of use and interpretation combined with resistance to drug effects make them an ideal choice not only for intraoperative monitoring, but also for monitoring and prognostication in the ICU. SSEPs are recorded by electrically stimulating a peripheral nerve (most commonly the median nerve at the wrist for upper limbs, the posterior tibial nerve at the ankle for lower limbs) and recording resulting responses at various levels rostrally. A brachial plexus peripheral nerve response is usually evident after only a few averages from an electrode at Erb's point. A spinal cord response can also be recorded after only a few averages from an electrode over the posterior neck. The cortical response usually requires 100 to 200 averages to produce a high-quality and consistent recording but may be evident more quickly in a completely relaxed, sedated ICU patient. A disruption in SSEPs can be caused by lesions in the peripheral nerve, spinal roots, spinal cord, brainstem, or cortex. Measuring a signal at each point along the way allows the electrophysiologist to confirm that the peripheral nerve has been stimulated successfully, rule out technical problems, and analyze and localize the level of dysfunction when responses are abnormal. The different waveforms reported on a SSEP recording are named after the direction of deflection (upward labeled as negative) and latency from the onset of stimulus in milliseconds (eg, N20 is the cortical response to upper limb stimulation, a negative polarity response which peaks at 20 ms). (See Figure 9.1 for an example of normal SSEPs.) Later responses can be seen in some subjects (eg, for the upper limb, a P30 and N70), which are typically more broadly distributed in the head, and are taken to indicate secondary cortical processing. Their variability between subjects, and absence in some normal patients, preclude routine clinical use (8,9).

Brainstem Auditory Evoked Potentials (BAEP)

Sound is the stimulus used in order to generate auditory evoked potentials. A series of clicks or tones are produced via headphones directly into the patient's ears, with resulting small electrical signals recorded from the scalp and ears. The signal generated in the cochlea travels through the cochlear nerve, into the superior olivary complex, up to the inferior colliculi, and through the medial geniculate bodies before reaching the cortex. Since most of these structures lie in the brainstem, this test can be used as a surrogate measure of brainstem integrity. In contrast to limb SSEPs, BAEPs require several hundred to a few thousand averages to generate a clear average. As for SSEPs, later responses, taken to indicate cortical response, can be recorded, but also are not generally clinically used due to variability.

Visual Evoked Potentials (VEP)

An evoked potential can be recorded from the occipital lobes when subjects are presented with visual stimuli. This test can be used to assess the primary visual pathways arising from the optic nerves and optic tracts extending through the lateral geniculate bodies, optic radiations, and to the occipital cortex. In routine clinical use, an alternating checkerboard visual stimulus is the most effective at producing a cortical response, however, this stimulus

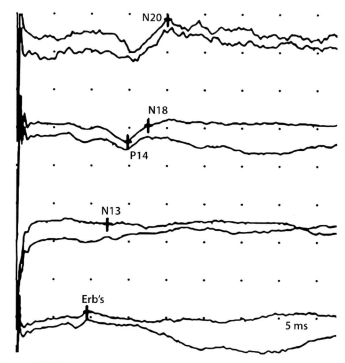

FIGURE 9.1 Normal SSEPs in response to stimulation of the median nerve at the wrist. Traces are displayed with the most caudal site at the bottom, the most rostral at the top. Two traces are performed at each level to verify consistently repeating responses. Traces show a degree of artifactual noise and baseline variability that is not atypical for the ICU environment, which is a considerably more electrically challenging environment than an electrically isolated outpatient neurophysiology laboratory. The traces demonstrate clearly preserved responses at all levels: Erb's point (the brachial plexus), the N13 response (cervical spinal cord), P14 and N18 (subcortical responses in the region of the foramen magnum), and the N20 (the primary somatosensory cerebral cortex).

requires an awake cooperative patient. Flash stimuli delivered with LED goggles can be used in uncooperative or cognitively impaired patients, but can only provide "all or nothing" characterization of function, and cannot rule in substantial but subtotal injury to the visual pathways.

PROGNOSIS AFTER CARDIAC ARREST

SSEPs have long been the most reliable, early electrophysiologic marker of poor prognosis after cardiac arrest (10). In these studies, the implicit mechanistic conclusion is that when the N20 response is absent, the anoxic injury experienced has been of sufficient severity to destroy the primary somatosensory cortico-neuronal pool (or the thalamic relay nuclei projecting to that pool). Clearly, it is not this system that is responsible for maintaining consciousness, but the implication is that similarly functionally devastating injury must have been experienced by those systems responsible for maintaining consciousness. Whatever the exact mechanism, absence of the short-latency N20 cortical response bilaterally to median nerve stimulation, when measured in the first 24 to 72 hours post–cardiac arrest, predicts poor prognosis (persistent coma or vegetative state). In a pivotal study of

305 comatose cardiac arrest patients, no false positives were observed (11). Robinson's 2003 meta-analysis of 18 studies involving 1,136 adult patients in hypoxic-ischemic coma showed no awakening in patients with absent cortical SSEP in follow-ups ranging from 1 month to 1 year (12). A more recent meta-analysis also confirms the ability of absent SSEP to predict poor outcomes, and also reports that it is marginally more accurate than the motor component of the Glasgow Coma Scale (GCS) (13). The 2006 guidelines from the American Academy of Neurology have affirmed the value of SSEP in prognostication of patients not treated with hypothermia (14). The 2008 Consensus Statement on Post Cardiac Arrest Syndrome and the 2010 Advanced Cardiac Life Support Guidelines of American Heart Association reaffirm the use in non hypothermia treated patients but provide caution on the use of SSEP in early prognostication in patients treated with hypothermia (15,16). Figure 9.2 presents an example of bilaterally absent N20 responses in a patient after cardiac arrest.

Conversely, the presence of the N20 response is not predictive of a good outcome. In Robinson's meta-analysis, presence of the N20 cortical responses, normal or abnormal, was associated with an awakening rate of 41%. Furthermore, in patients with normal SSEP responses, the awakening rate was still only 52% (12). The low predictive value of present N20 responses is probably in part due to the fact that short-latency responses only test for an intact primary somatosensory pathway, most of which lie in subcortical structures. More complex cortical–cortical and thalamocortical interactions are needed to maintain consciousness (17,18).

Long-latency SSEP responses, such as the N70, have also been studied in order to improve the positive predictive value of SSEP for good outcomes as they should represent these cortical–cortical responses. One such study of 162 unconscious patients resuscitated from cardiac arrest published in 2000 showed the N70 latency had high sensitivity (94%) and specificity (97%) for favorable outcomes using a cutoff of presence prior to 130 ms (19). A subsequent small study also supported good predictive value of the long-latency responses (20). However, a later study of 319 patients did not reproduce the same robust results when using a N70 latency cutoff of 130 ms as a prognostic marker (21). The use of long-latency SSEPs in this setting remains contentious.

Other EP modalities are less well characterized for use in evaluating postanoxic coma patients. Guerit et al evaluated the prognostic value of BAEPs and flash VEPs along with concurrent SSEP (22). The contribution from BAEPs for prognosis was only apparent in a stratified combination of the other two testing modalities, and was meaningfully contributory in their scheme only when SSEPs were absent at the cortical level. At this level, the absence of a BAEP response was predictive of an even more consistently dismal prognosis than preserved BAEP with severely abnormal SSEP. Another study evaluating SSEP and BAEP reported that BAEP waveform analysis was not helpful when used alone or in combination with the SSEP in determining prognosis after cardiac arrest (23). On close review of their text, of the four patients in whom no such analysis was possible due to absence of the BAEP altogether, three of them never regained consciousness. Collectively, reported numbers of patients with absent BAEP responses in case series of postanoxic comatose patients is low. While the significance of absent BAEP is consistently dismal, there are insufficient numbers reported in any one series to permit utilization of the test with the same level of confidence as with SSEPs. It is

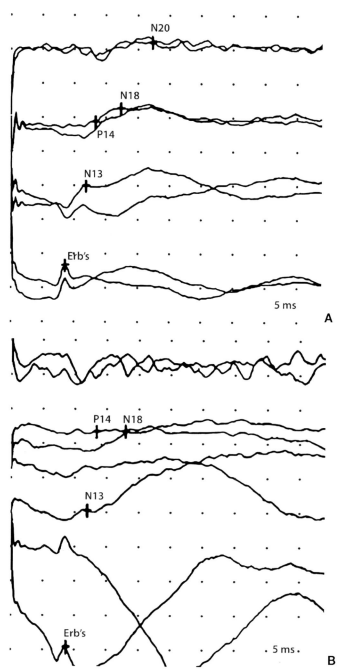

FIGURE 9.2 Example of abnormal SSEPs with absent bilateral N20 responses in a patient after cardiac arrest. Both A (left arm stimulation) and B (right) show clearly preserved Erb's point and N13 responses—an important finding, as this establishes that stimulation was performed in a technically correct fashion, and verifies residual peripheral nerve and spinal cord function. Part B demonstrates no clear repeating response at either the subcortical or cortical level, and would likely be interpreted by most physiologists as an absent response. Part A suggests a preserved subcortical response; at the cortical level, there is a downward deflection at 15 ms, but no repeating response thereafter—this is a challenging record, and would likely be interpreted as absent by many physiologists, but could be interpreted as low amplitude but preserved response by others.

tempting to conclude that the absence of these patients with abnormal BAEPs from the literature is precisely because patients with poor outcome do not survive long enough to be included in BAEP studies. This must remain a speculation, however, and all that can be said with a high degree of confidence is that neither BAEPs nor flash VEPs can be utilized for prognostication in the same evidence-based fashion as SSEPs.

An important consideration in the utilization of EPs for prognostication in coma is noise level. High levels of electrical noise from medical equipment are not uncommon when recording in ICU environments and render SSEP recordings more difficult to confidently interpret. This results in significantly lower inter rater reliabilities (24). ICUs that wish to incorporate EP recordings into the evaluation of comatose patients may benefit from disconnecting as many electrical devices from the patient as possible during recording times.

A more recent consideration is the effect of therapeutic hypothermia on the validity of SSEP for prognostication. A meta-analysis of 1,153 patients evaluated the effect of hypothermia on prognostic markers after cardiac arrest and reported the false-positive rate of bilaterally absent N20s as still less than 1% (25). While some recent smaller studies on SSEP recorded during therapeutic hypothermia appear to retain its good prognostic value in predicting poor outcomes, it is important to note that these studies have a large proportion of patients die as a consequence of withdrawal of life-sustaining therapies (26,27). Lack of total blinding of the clinicians to the prognostic test result opens these studies to a high possibility of self-fulfilling prophecies (28,29).

PROGNOSIS AFTER TRAUMATIC BRAIN INJURY

The use of EPs for determination of neurologic prognosis after traumatic brain injury (TBI) has been well studied. One earlier study looked at the predictive value of SSEP in comatose TBI patients (30). The authors evaluated 51 unresponsive, intubated patients using median nerve SSEP within 1 week after initial injury. The SSEPs were assigned a grade of 1 to 6 (1 = absent cortical responses, 6 = normal cortical responses), and the clinical outcome was measured using the Glasgow Outcome Scale and Barthel Index at 6 months. All patients with SSEP Grade 1 died or remained in a vegetative state, and no SSEP Grade 2 patient improved beyond severe disability. Conversely, all patients with SSEP Grade 6 had good recoveries or at most moderate disability (30). The same SSEP grading scale was also used to demonstrate prognostic value for functional and cognitive outcomes after 1 year. The SSEP grade on Day 3 after head injury displayed the strongest correlation with 1 year functional and cognitive measures (31).

In a meta-analysis of 14 studies incorporating 838 comatose adult and teenage patients with TBI, SSEP was demonstrated to have fairly good predictive value (12). Patients who had absent bilateral SSEP (generally meaning absent N20 responses) progressed to death or persistent vegetative state 95% of the time. Patients with normal SSEPs improved to good recovery and moderate disability 57% and 22% of the time, respectively. Although the predictive value of SSEP is good in the setting of TBI, the data suggest that approximately 1 in 20 patients with initially absent SSEP will still ultimately awaken, most with severe disability (12). This is considerably higher than the awakening rate of patients with hypoxic-ischemic coma. The addition of other sensory EP modalities (BAEP, VEP) or including long-latency responses does not significantly alter the prognostic value (32). Nevertheless, when compared to other clinical tests such as GCS, EEG, or CT, SSEP may have the potential to be the best single overall predictor of neurologic outcomes (33).

PROGNOSIS AFTER ISCHEMIC OR HEMORRHAGIC STROKE

EPs have also been used for determining prognosis in settings of ischemic or hemorrhagic stroke, although this has been much less studied. A study of 70 comatose patients after subarachnoid or hypertensive hemorrhages found that AEP and SSEP had high sensitivity and specificity in predicting neurologic outcomes, but not at the level of certainty necessary for accurate prognostication (34). Robinson's meta-analysis of 157 patients with intracerebral hemorrhage showed more predictive results to some extent with only 1% (confidence interval [CI] 0%–4%) awakening if SSEP was absent (12). However, the number of patients included in the study remains too low to allow the routine use of SSEP for determining prognosis in this setting.

Few studies have looked at the ability of EPs to predict outcomes in severe ischemic strokes. One report on 84 patients with large hemispheric strokes demonstrated high specificity and predictive value for poor outcomes if there was bilateral absence of SSEP N20 and BAEP Wave V, though the sensitivity remained low (35).

PROGNOSIS AFTER SPINAL CORD INJURY

Studies have also shown that SSEP can be used to help distinguish patients with good versus poor chances of recovery from spinal cord injury. In one study looking at 36 patients in the early weeks after acute cervical cord injury, the investigators discovered that patients with absent cortical responses had much worse outcomes than those with present cortical responses. This finding was useful in patients with incomplete neurologic injury that could not be clinically separated by neurologic exam alone. All the patients with complete functional loss had absent cortical responses (36). A more recent study also demonstrated that early presence of tibial SSEPs after spinal cord injury was associated with favorable neurologic recoveries, although the converse was not always true (37). Furthermore, additional studies also confirm the prognostic value of EPs during initial treatment phases and advocate for their use in planning appropriate rehabilitation regimens (38,39).

PROGNOSIS FOR METABOLIC ENCEPHALOPATHY

Few studies have looked at the utility of EPs in the setting of other forms of encephalopathy such as septic or hepatic encephalopathy. One study on metabolic encephalopathy reported a direct correlation between the degree of cortical SSEP peak latencies and the severity of patients' critical illness as measured by Acute Physiology and Chronic Health Evaluation III scores (APACHE III) (40). A subsequent study showed the prevalence of septic encephalopathy as measured by prolonged SSEP is higher than generally assumed (41).

Multimodal EP abnormalities have been reported to be detectable even before the onset of clinically apparent hepatic encephalopathy (42). The disappearance of short latency cortical potentials in patients with severe hepatic encephalopathies has also been reported to be an ominous sign heralding increased intracranial pressure (ICP) and death (43).

CONTINUOUS EVOKED POTENTIAL MONITORING IN THE NEUROLOGIC ICU

Despite the proven prognostic value of EPs in patients with severe brain injury, there have been few studies on the use of continuous evoked potential (CEP) monitoring. Only two groups in the literature have studied this method rigorously (44,45).

The first group monitored 65 patients with severe closed head injuries using SSEP concurrently with ICP and arterial–jugular oxygen content difference (AVDO2) monitoring (44). They found that 89% of patients with absent long-latency (greater than 50 ms) responses either died or were vegetative at 3 months. All patients with preserved N70 or later responses had good or moderate outcomes. Furthermore, they found that deteriorations in the SSEP signal correlated with drops in AVDO2, but not with increases in ICP (44). Subsequently, this group compared CEP with continuous EEG monitoring in 103 patients with severe closed head injuries. Patients were monitored on average for 5 days, until they regained consciousness, died, or were declared to be clinically stable. They discovered the CEP was much better at detecting changes in neurologic condition than the continuous EEG monitoring, especially on sedated and paralyzed patients (6).

The second study was successful in detecting neurologic deterioration early by using CEP (45). They studied a cohort of 68 patients with head trauma and intracranial hemorrhage with continuous SSEP and EEG monitoring. Patients who were stable or improving did not show any significant changes in their SSEPs. However, in all 13 patients who deteriorated neurologically, SSEPs showed disappearance or significant alterations in amplitude. The alterations in amplitude were progressive decreases or paradoxical increases preceding disappearance of the potentials. This group also found significant correlation with the patients' ICPs, with SSEP deterioration preceding ICP increase in 30% of patients. Particularly, the authors pointed out the helpfulness of the SSEP in patients with ICP ranging 20 to 40 mmHg, as these patients could not be reliably predicted to deteriorate despite their abnormally high ICP (45). With increasing evidence questioning the long-cherished validity of ICP monitoring, SSEP monitoring offers an alternative that is based more on function (46). Finally, they found the SSEP monitoring to be more informative than the EEG as many of their patients were sedated (45).

Although studies are sparse on continuous EP monitoring in patients with severe neurologic injury, it is reasonable to consider this approach in patients in whom a neurologic exam cannot be consistently followed, such as those who are ventilated, sedated, and/or paralyzed. With further study, repeated performance of EPs may ultimately become an essential part of multimodality monitoring in the neurologic ICU.

FUTURE DIRECTIONS

The adoption and use of EPs in clinical practice are predicated on the notion that we understand well the underlying mechanisms of normal and abnormal signals. However, beyond the few named potentials mentioned herein, there is not widespread agreement on the exact origin or significance of these waveforms (47,48). In animal studies of cardiac arrest, insights into the significance of specific components of the SSEP are revealing new prospects for research (49). Moreover, while current use of SSEPs often rely on a dichotomized system of present or absent responses at specific time intervals, new research has shown a clear evolution of the signal during recovery from cardiac arrest that is amenable to quantitative analysis useful for prognostication (49,50). The future of EP monitoring in the neurological ICU lies in our ability to understand and recognize the subtle changes in a dynamic signal, and to harness that information to apply effective clinical care.

REFERENCES

1. Desmedt JE, Huy NT, Bourguet M. The cognitive P40, N60 and P100 components of somatosensory evoked potentials and the earliest electrical signs of sensory processing in man. *Electroencephalography and clinical neurophysiology.* 1983 Oct; 56(4):272–282. PubMed PMID: 6193940.

2. Hayashi N, Nishijo H, Ono T, et al. Generators of somatosensory evoked potentials investigated by dipole tracing in the monkey. *Neuroscience.* 1995 Sep; 68(2):323–338. PubMed PMID: 7477944. Epub 1995/09/01. eng.

3. Hillyard SA, Kutas M. Electrophysiology of cognitive processing. *Annual review of psychology.* 1983;34:33–61. PubMed PMID: 6338812.

4. McPherson RW, Sell B, Traystman RJ. Effects of thiopental, fentanyl, and etomidate on upper extremity somatosensory evoked potentials in humans. *Anesthesiology.* 1986 Dec; 65(6):584–589. PubMed PMID: 3789431.

5. Drummond JC, Todd MM, U HS. The effect of high dose sodium thiopental on brain stem auditory and median nerve somatosensory evoked responses in humans. *Anesthesiology.* 1985 Sep; 63(3):249–254. PubMed PMID: 4025886.

6. Moulton RJ, Brown JI, Konasiewicz SJ. Monitoring severe head injury: a comparison of EEG and somatosensory evoked potentials. *The Canadian journal of neurological sciences/Le journal canadien des sciences neurologiques.* 1998 Feb; 25(1):S7–S11. PubMed PMID: 9532290.

7. Vincent A. Methods for improving the signal-to-noise ratio of endogenous-evoked potentials. Integrative physiological and behavioral science: The official journal of the Pavlovian Society. 1992 Jan–Mar; 27(1):54–65. PubMed PMID: 1576088.

8. Huisman UW, Posthuma J, Hooijer C, et al. Somatosensory evoked potentials in healthy volunteers and in patients with dementia. *Clinical neurology and neurosurgery.* 1985;87(1):11–16. PubMed PMID: 3987136.

9. Colon EJ, de Weerd AW. Long-latency somatosensory evoked potentials. *Journal of clinical neurophysiology: official publication of the American Electroencephalographic Society.* 1986 Oct; 3(4):279–296. PubMed PMID: 3332278.

10. Young GB. Clinical practice. Neurologic prognosis after cardiac arrest. *The New England journal of medicine.* 2009 Aug 6; 361(6):605–611. PubMed PMID: 19657124. Epub 2009/08/07. eng.

11. Zandbergen EG, Hijdra A, Koelman JH, et al. Prediction of poor outcome within the first 3 days of postanoxic coma. *Neurology.* 2006 Jan 10; 66(1):62–68. PubMed PMID: 16401847.

12. Robinson LR, Micklesen PJ, Tirschwell DL, Lew HL. Predictive value of somatosensory evoked potentials for awakening from coma. *Critical care medicine.* 2003 Mar; 31(3):960–967. PubMed PMID: 12627012.

13. Lee YC, Phan TG, Jolley DJ, et al. Accuracy of clinical signs, SEP, and EEG in predicting outcome of hypoxic coma: a meta-analysis. *Neurology.* 2010 Feb 16; 74(7):572–580. PubMed PMID: 20157159.

14. Wijdicks EF, Hijdra A, Young GB, et al. Practice parameter: prediction of outcome in comatose survivors after cardiopulmonary resuscitation (an evidence-based review): report of the Quality Standards Subcommittee of the American Academy of Neurology. *Neurology.* 2006 Jul 25; 67(2):203–210. PubMed PMID: 16864809. Epub 2006/07/26. eng.

15. Neumar RW, Nolan JP, Adrie C, et al. Post-cardiac arrest syndrome: epidemiology, pathophysiology, treatment, and prognostication. A consensus statement from the International Liaison Committee on Resuscitation (American Heart Association, Australian and New Zealand Council on Resuscitation, European Resuscitation Council, Heart and Stroke Foundation of Canada, InterAmerican Heart Foundation, Resuscitation Council of Asia, and the Resuscitation Council of Southern Africa); the American Heart Association Emergency Cardiovascular Care Committee; the Council on Cardiovascular Surgery and Anesthesia; the Council on Cardiopulmonary, Perioperative, and Critical Care; the Council on Clinical Cardiology; and the Stroke Council. *Circulation.* 2008 Dec 2; 118(23): 2452–2483. PubMed PMID: 18948368. Epub 2008/10/25. eng.

16. Peberdy MA, Callaway CW, Neumar RW, et al. Part 9: post-cardiac arrest care: 2010 American Heart Association Guidelines for Cardiopulmonary Resuscitation and Emergency Cardiovascular Care. *Circulation*. 2010 Nov 2; 122(18 Suppl 3):S768–S786. PubMed PMID: 20956225.

17. John ER. The neurophysics of consciousness. *Brain research—Brain research reviews*. 2002 Jun; 39(1):1–28. PubMed PMID: 12086706.

18. Llinas R, Ribary U, Contreras D, Pedroarena C. The neuronal basis for consciousness. Philosophical transactions of the Royal Society of London Series B, Biological sciences. 1998 Nov 29; 353(1377): 1841–1849. PubMed PMID: 9854256. Pubmed Central PMCID: 1692417. Epub 1998/12/17. eng.

19. Madl C, Kramer L, Domanovits H, et al. Improved outcome prediction in unconscious cardiac arrest survivors with sensory evoked potentials compared with clinical assessment. *Critical care medicine*. 2000 Mar; 28(3):721–726. PubMed PMID: 10752821.

20. Young GB, Doig G, Ragazzoni A. Anoxic-ischemic encephalopathy: clinical and electrophysiological associations with outcome. *Neurocrit Care*. 2005;2(2):159–164. PubMed PMID: 16159058. Epub 2005/09/15. eng.

21. Zandbergen EG, Koelman JH, de Haan RJ, et al. Group PR-S. SSEPs and prognosis in postanoxic coma: only short or also long latency responses? *Neurology*. 2006 Aug 22; 67(4):583–586. PubMed PMID: 16924008.

22. Guerit JM, de Tourtchaninoff M, Soveges L, et al. The prognostic value of three-modality evoked potentials (TMEPs) in anoxic and traumatic comas. *Neurophysiologie clinique [Clinical neurophysiology]*. 1993 May; 23(2–3):209–226. PubMed PMID: 8326931.

23. Tiainen M, Kovala TT, Takkunen OS, et al. Somatosensory and brainstem auditory evoked potentials in cardiac arrest patients treated with hypothermia. *Critical care medicine*. 2005 Aug; 33(8):1736–1740. PubMed PMID: 16096450.

24. Zandbergen EG, Hijdra A, de Haan RJ, et al. Interobserver variation in the interpretation of SSEPs in anoxic-ischaemic coma. *Clinical neurophysiology: official journal of the International Federation of Clinical Neurophysiology*. 2006 Jul; 117(7):1529–1535. PubMed PMID: 16697253.

25. Kamps MJ, Horn J, Oddo M, et al. Prognostication of neurologic outcome in cardiac arrest patients after mild therapeutic hypothermia: a meta-analysis of the current literature. *Intensive care medicine*. 2013 Jun 26. PubMed PMID: 23801384.

26. Grippo A, Carrai R, Fossi S, et al. Absent SEP during therapeutic hypothermia did not reappear after re-warming in comatose patients following cardiac arrest. *Minerva anestesiologica*. 2013 Apr; 79(4):360–369. PubMed PMID: 23449240.

27. Bouwes A, Binnekade JM, Zandstra DF, et al. Somatosensory evoked potentials during mild hypothermia after cardiopulmonary resuscitation. *Neurology*. 2009 Nov 3; 73(18):1457–1461. PubMed PMID: 19884573.

28. Geocadin RG, Kaplan PW. Neural repair and rehabilitation: the effect of therapeutic hypothermia on prognostication. *Nature reviews Neurology*. 2012 Jan; 8(1):5–6. PubMed PMID: 22198403.

29. Kalanuria AA, Geocadin RG. Early prognostication in acute brain damage: where is the evidence? *Current opinion in critical care*. 2013 Apr; 19(2):113–122. PubMed PMID: 23422160.

30. Houlden DA, Li C, Schwartz ML, et al. Median nerve somatosensory evoked potentials and the Glasgow Coma Scale as predictors of outcome in comatose patients with head injuries. *Neurosurgery*. 1990 Nov; 27(5):701–707; discussion 7–8. PubMed PMID: 2259399.

31. Houlden DA, Taylor AB, Feinstein A, et al. Early somatosensory evoked potential grades in comatose traumatic brain injury patients predict cognitive and functional outcome. *Critical care medicine*. 2010 Jan; 38(1):167–174. PubMed PMID: 19829103.

32. Kane NM, Curry SH, Rowlands CA, et al. Event-related potentials—neurophysiological tools for predicting emergence and early outcome from traumatic coma. *Intensive care medicine*. 1996 Jan; 22(1):39–46. PubMed PMID: 8857436.

33. Carter BG, Butt W. Are somatosensory evoked potentials the best predictor of outcome after severe brain injury? A systematic review. *Intensive care medicine*. 2005 Jun; 31(6):765–775. PubMed PMID: 15846481.

34. Facco E, Behr AU, Munari M, et al. Auditory and somatosensory evoked potentials in coma following spontaneous cerebral hemorrhage: early prognosis and outcome. *Electroencephalography and clinical neurophysiology*. 1998 Nov; 107(5):332–338. PubMed PMID: 9872435.

35. Zhang Y, Su YY, Haupt WF, et al. Application of electrophysiologic techniques in poor outcome prediction among patients with severe focal and diffuse ischemic brain injury. *Journal of clinical neurophysiology: Official publication of the American Electroencephalographic Society.* 2011 Oct; 28(5):497–503. PubMed PMID: 21946368.

36. Li C, Houlden DA, Rowed DW. Somatosensory evoked potentials and neurological grades as predictors of outcome in acute spinal cord injury. *Journal of neurosurgery.* 1990 Apr; 72(4):600–609. PubMed PMID: 2319320.

37. Spiess M, Schubert M, Kliesch U, group E-SS, Halder P. Evolution of tibial SSEP after traumatic spinal cord injury: baseline for clinical trials. *Clinical neurophysiology: official journal of the International Federation of Clinical Neurophysiology.* 2008 May; 119(5):1051–1061. PubMed PMID: 18343719.

38. Curt A, Dietz V. Electrophysiological recordings in patients with spinal cord injury: significance for predicting outcome. *Spinal cord.* 1999 Mar; 37(3):157–165. PubMed PMID: 10213324.

39. Curt A, Dietz V. Ambulatory capacity in spinal cord injury: significance of somatosensory evoked potentials and ASIA protocol in predicting outcome. *Archives of physical medicine and rehabilitation.* 1997 Jan; 78(1):39–43. PubMed PMID: 9014955.

40. Zauner C, Gendo A, Kramer L, et al. Metabolic encephalopathy in critically ill patients suffering from septic or nonseptic multiple organ failure. *Critical care medicine.* 2000 May; 28(5):1310–1315. PubMed PMID: 10834671.

41. Zauner C, Gendo A, Kramer L, et al. Impaired subcortical and cortical sensory evoked potential pathways in septic patients. *Critical care medicine.* 2002 May; 30(5):1136N1139. PubMed PMID: 12006815.

42. Ryu N, Gao W, Yan M. [Evaluation of brain evoked potentials in the detection of subclinical hepatic encephalopathy in cirrhotics]. *No to shinkei [Brain and nerve].* 1997 Oct; 49(10):887–892. PubMed PMID: 9368885.

43. Yang SS, Chu NS, Wu CH. Disappearance of N20 and P25 components of somatosensory evoked potential: an ominous sign in severe acute hepatitis. *Journal of the Formosan Medical Association [Taiwan yi zhi].* 1993 Jan; 92(1):46–49. PubMed PMID: 8099826.

44. Moulton RJ, Shedden PM, Tucker WS, et al. Somatosensory evoked potential monitoring following severe closed head injury. *Clinical and investigative medicine Medecine clinique et experimentale.* 1994 Jun; 17(3):187–195. PubMed PMID: 7923995.

45. Amantini A, Fossi S, Grippo A, et al. Continuous EEG-SEP monitoring in severe brain injury. *Neurophysiologie clinique [Clinical neurophysiology].* 2009 Apr; 39(2):85–93. PubMed PMID: 19467438.

46. Chesnut RM, Temkin N, Carney N, et al. A trial of intracranial-pressure monitoring in traumatic brain injury. *The New England journal of medicine.* 2012 Dec 27; 367(26):2471–2481. PubMed PMID: 23234472. Pubmed Central PMCID: 3565432.

47. Ulas UH, Ozdag F, Eroglu E, et al. Median nerve somatosensory evoked potentials recorded with cephalic and noncephalic references in central and peripheral nervous system lesions. *Clinical EEG.* 2001 Oct; 32(4):191–196. PubMed PMID: 11682813.

48. Buchner H, Fuchs M, Wischmann HA, et al. Source analysis of median nerve and finger stimulated somatosensory evoked potentials: multichannel simultaneous recording of electric and magnetic fields combined with 3D-MR tomography. *Brain topography.* 1994 Summer; 6(4):299–310. PubMed PMID: 7946929.

49. Xiong W, Koenig MA, Madhok J, et al. Evolution of Somatosensory Evoked Potentials after Cardiac Arrest induced hypoxic-ischemic injury. *Resuscitation.* 2010 Jul; 81(7):893–897. PubMed PMID: 20418008. Pubmed Central PMCID: 2893290. Epub 2010/04/27. eng.

50. Madhok J, Maybhate A, Xiong W, et al. Quantitative assessment of somatosensory-evoked potentials after cardiac arrest in rats: prognostication of functional outcomes. *Critical care medicine.* 2010 Aug; 38(8):1709–1717. PubMed PMID: 20526197. Pubmed Central PMCID: 3050516. Epub 2010/06/08. eng.

Bioinformatics for Multimodal Monitoring

J. Michael Schmidt, PhD, MSc

INTRODUCTION

The goal of invasive neuromonitoring, or multimodality monitoring, is to provide neuro-physiologic decision support at the bedside. Advanced monitoring techniques can provide real-time information regarding the relative health or distress of the brain. This information can be used to detect the onset of secondary brain injuries that may be intervened upon and to set physiologic end points to guide goal-directed therapy and thereby create and maintain an optimal physiologic environment for the comatose injured brain to heal (1). It is now practical to store huge volumes of patient neuromonitoring data, but additional work is required in order to integrate it with other patient care information to enable the extraction of clinically useful information hidden within it.

Clinical informatics, a subfield of biomedical informatics, deals with biomedical information, data, and knowledge including their storage, retrieval, and optimal use for problem solving and decision making as applied to problems in clinical care (2). Clinical informatics, as an interdisciplinary field, utilizes a wide range of statistical, signal processing, pattern recognition, machine learning, and visualization tools to support data analysis and discovery of important information and patterns embedded within medical data repositories (2,3). This is a growing field that will have a tremendous impact on medicine in general and intensive care unit (ICU) care in particular where high-frequency, high-volume medical data are most available.

Multimodality Monitoring as Translational Research

According to the National Institutes of Health roadmap, the goal of translational research is to translate scientific discovery that typically begins at "the bench" into practical applications that progress to the clinical level, or the patient's "bedside" (4). Translational multimodality monitoring uses a less common bedside-to-bench model and presents unique challenges. This research model is less established because it is often poorly understood by full-time clinicians, unappreciated by basic scientists, and greeted by an unsympathetic review process (5). Building a two-way (bedside-to-bench-to-bedside) translational clinical informatics infrastructure for multimodality monitoring is vital to its long-term success.

Multimodality monitoring two-way translational research is made up of four interdependent elements or steps that together compose a translational research platform. Each step has its own unique challenges that must be met. The first step is to acquire and store all relevant data into a single database, data repository, or enterprise-level clinical data warehouse. Creating the informatics infrastructure for this is a major focus of this chapter. Second, clinically relevant features must be extracted from the raw data and converted into clinical information. This step requires infrastructure to process data with a wide range of analysis tools spanning many scientific disciplines (6). These two steps represent bedside-to-bench research, whereas the next two steps are bench-to-bedside research. The third step is to take actionable clinical information and present it at the bedside in a manner that provides clinicians situational awareness of patient status or changes in patient state (7). Ideally, new kinds of information can be evaluated at the bedside through a clinical study. Multimodality monitoring is a step toward personalized medicine and as such it is not a rare occurrence to be confronted by data from a specific patient that suggest taking actions that are not in alignment with evidence-based protocols. The last step then is for clinical information gleaned from multimodality monitoring determined as valuable to be integrated into clinical practice and workflow (Chapter 10).

Cohen et al (8) conducted a bedside-to-bench study by applying a hierarchical clustering algorithm to 1-minute resolution multimodal physiologic and ventilator data. Each of the ten clusters produced were then correlated with outcome measures. It was found that patients spent significant time in different clusters, and transitions between clusters (ie, patient states) were detectable. Most importantly the analysis revealed patient states associated with mortality that were not recognizable to clinicians. This study demonstrates that there are patterns embedded within multimodality data that require analysis to extract, and highlights the tremendous potential of multimodality monitoring translational research.

The study by Cohen et al (8) is an exemplar of half of the translational research cycle. Hypothetically the investigators could conduct a follow-up study to test whether a specific intervention could alter a patient state associated with mortality to a patient state associated with survival. Barriers to conducting such a study are important to articulate. From a clinical-informatics standpoint, the ability to conduct the study rests on the capability to apply one's algorithms to high resolution physiologic data and deliver the results to the bedside in real time. This point is crucial because the informatics infrastructure required to conduct real-time analysis and display are essential to fully complete the translational research cycle.

There are content barriers as well that are true for many aspect of neuromonitoring research. For example, Bardt et al (9) showed in TBI that $P_{bt}O_2$ less than 10 mmHg for 10 minutes was associated with increased risk of death. We know of several ways to increase $P_{bt}O_2$ (10), but this does not imply that "improving" $P_{bt}O_2$ will necessarily alleviate this risk.

If we presume that the patient states revealed in Cohen et al (8) are less understood than $P_{bt}O_2$, then investigators would have to first study the underlying patient states to determine if they were modifiable by treatment, and if so, by what means. Each patient state would need to have a clinical hypothesis that provided a rationale for intervention. Only then could a series of intervention studies be devised. In short, what began as a bedside-to-bench study would shift to bench-to-bedside research. Each phase of research has unique challenges and requires different skill sets. Multimodality monitoring research requires clinical investigators to be adept at both and highlights why multidisciplinary, and perhaps multi-institutional, research teams are appealing.

Research from the neonatal ICU provides a good example of effective bedside-to-bench-to-bedside translational research. Investigators hypothesized that heart rate variability monitoring could be used to identify preclinical stages of sepsis in neonates. Bedside data were collected from the physiologic monitor and heart rate variability algorithms trained to identify sepsis risk were developed in the computer lab (11,12). The team built a monitoring device that could process real-time EKG and produce their algorithm results at the bedside. In a randomized clinical trial they reported a 20% infant mortality benefit in patients when the monitor was used (13). This was a substantial but necessary effort that the field of multimodal neuromonitoring must emulate in order to make progress.

PHYSIOLOGICAL DATA COLLECTION

General Considerations

There are several considerations before investing in high resolution data acquisition for a translational neuromonitoring platform. A significant amount of time is required to collect, manipulate, and analyze high-resolution patient data. These data will most likely need to be stored in a separate database and then combined with other study data. For epidemiologic and other clinical studies, data reduction methods will be required to reduce its frequency to a resolution (eg, hours) amenable to standard biostatistical approaches. For these kinds of studies, it may be more efficient and in most cases sufficient to collect hourly data from an electronic medical record. Indeed many meaningful studies can be performed without high-resolution physiologic data. Thought should be given to whether its collection will be beneficial to a research program or unnecessarily burdensome.

Hospital Collaboration

Hospital administrators may be focused on electronic health record (EHR) adoption and may not consider high-resolution physiologic data a high priority. One strategy can be to collaborate with hospital quality control teams to address problems they are interested in solving, such as creating the infrastructure needed to intervene and impact patient outcomes and length of stay. This same infrastructure will also support your translational research program. It is also noteworthy that many aspects of clinical informatics systems for the ICU will require hospital support. There may be network and storage concerns or purchased equipment will need to maintained over time and require a long-term budget. The hospital will also control access to other critical data in the EHR. Developing a relationship with hospital teams will be beneficial in the long term.

Data Acquistion Challenges

A typical neuromonitoring patient will have a host of devices attached including cardio-pulmonary monitors, a ventilator, brain monitoring equipment including EEG, perhaps a cooling device, and numerous infusion pumps. Many devices will plug into the bedside physiologic monitor, but many devices will not or do so incompletely (ie, not all important data are transferred). Medical device connectivity is complex because each device can have a different physical connector and use its own communication protocol to transfer its data. Simply associating device data to a patient can be a technical challenge depending on the method of data acquisition. Infusion pumps should have the capability to send streaming data, yet not all do, and of those that do some only transmit anonymous drug and dose data. Synchronizing data in time from multiple devices may also be challenging because a device may maintain its own internal clock. Integrating such data together requires knowing the actual time so that they can be fused properly.

Fortunately numerous commercial products exist to address these issues and options improve every year. But in evaluating them it is important to understand how each system handles these issues and what the limitations are. For example, the General Electric 8000i monitor, collected parameters are labeled with the designation selected by the nurse plus the port number it is plugged into on the monitor. If a patient has an ICP monitor plugged into port 3, then they label would be ICP3 for instance. It is not uncommon for neuromonitoring patients to have both an endoventricular drain (EVD) and parenchymal ICP monitor at the same time. If the EVD is plugged into port 3 and the parenchymal monitor is plugged into port 5, then they would be ICP3 and ICP5, respectively. When the patient is taken for a procedure or scan, everything will be unplugged, and upon the patient's return it is not guaranteed that the EVD will be plugged back into port 3 and the parenchymal monitor into port 5. In fact, often that will not be the case, and these monitors will have new labels or, worse, the same labels in reverse (ie, the EVD is now ICP5). This implementation works if one is only viewing the last 5 seconds of data on the bedside monitor, but when trying to analyze the last 3 days of data, it becomes very difficult to discern which data correspond to which device. Every commercial system has tradeoffs, but this highlights some of the potentially unexpected difficulties in working with high-resolution data.

Data Frequency and Storage Requirements

Some thought should also go into what specific frequency data should be collected and stored. Unfortunately, there is no clear guideline for this. For some applications, data collected every 10 minutes can be sufficient whereas for cerebral autoregulation indices (14) data collected every 5 seconds is needed. Waveform data are usually available at the frequency used by the patient monitor or device. Storing data at the highest frequency possible is probably the most prudent course. In our neurologic ICU, we store approximately 200 megabytes (MB)/day/bed collecting, 5-sec resolution digital data into a SQL database and 2-sec resolution digital data plus 240 Hz waveform data into individual binary files. Continuous EEG recordings can generate approximately 1 gigabyte (GB)/day for EEG alone, and 20 GB/day when including video.

If these data travel over the hospital network, IT administrators will want to ensure that ethernet networks employ 1 GB/sec or greater connections between switches and routers to avoid network performance slowdowns or data loss (15). In some institutions as a matter of policy, high-resolution patient data are erased several months after discharge unless there is a specific request to save it. For translational research, it is critical to permanently store data in a data warehouse for current and future projects. The value of annotated high-resolution physiologic data to translational research cannot be overstated and if the effort is going to be made to collect it, it should be saved. Optimally, physiologic data should be stored using a standard open format that can be utilized by any number of viewing or analysis systems.

Physiological Data Acquisition Approaches

Broadly there are two basic approaches to acquire and store high-resolution data. One can either monitor a few selected patients at a time using portable carts that can be moved from room to room, or have a fixed system that monitors all patient beds simultaneously. The "right" approach will depend on the particular situation of an institution. Purchasing a portable cart and moving it to the room from which you wish to collect monitoring data is akin to purchasing a medical device. These commercially available systems take data directly from the patient monitor and peripheral devices in order to display the data on its screen.

There are several conveniences to this strategy. For clinical purposes, these devices provide a limited set of patient-specific analyses that are performed and presented to clinicians in real time at the bedside. They also tend to be easy to use by clinical staff and easy to maintain, and hospitals have established administrative processes to purchase ICU devices and, therefore, their purchase is likely the quickest path to implementing a live system in the ICU. This may be a particularly appealing option if one is looking to add both EEG and neuromonitoring to the ICU.

There are several tradeoffs, however, that impact both long-term clinical utility and research. First, the data acquired may or may not be stored into an open database format. Clinically, this will mean that it will be very difficult to use the data in any way other than how it is analyzed and presented on the device screen. This is mitigated somewhat if the device provides a mechanism for real-time export to other systems. In the absence of open data availability, it will be difficult to integrate the acquired data with data in other hospital clinical information systems. The data storage format also affects archiving the data for clinical research purposes, which may prove to be cumbersome and may not lend itself to group analysis. Neuromonitoring carts are FDA approved and priced like an expensive medical device. The cost of purchasing two or three carts can, in many cases, pay for whole ICU data acquisition from the physiologic monitor. The cost–benefit ratio of purchasing a cart-based solution is probably only realized if the system provides acquisition and integration of both EEG and neuromonitoring data.

The second approach is to simultaneously collect all patient physiologic monitor and neuromonitoring device data and store them on an enterprise level central server (16,17). A server is simply a class of computers with large computational and storage capacities that manage, store, and retrieve data for other computers or devices (18). The central server will need to be operated and supported over time, which is an expense that must be budgeted for and most likely supported by hospital IT. It is important to assess the extent to which hospital administrators and IT understand and are committed to neurophysiologic decision support in the ICU—this is an essential prerequisite before considering purchasing ICU-wide solutions.

EEG Data Collection and Research

Kull and Emerson (19) cover in detail general considerations related to EEG monitoring in the ICU. EEG integration with other modalities is beginning to become more feasible. EKG signal acquisition onto EEG systems allows potential integration of it with other modalities by synchronizing two separate data streams by the common EKG signal. In practice, though integrating EEG waveform and bedside physiology acquired in separate systems remains painful. Quantitative EEG (qEEG) can usually be manually exported and connected to other modalities for research. For clinical research, this is more or less acceptable but fails to address the larger question of translational research since there is currently no good way to evaluate new discoveries for its clinical utility at the bedside.

Translational Research Integrating High Resolution Data with EEG

A recently published bedside-to-bench study (20) highlights some of the challenges of and opportunities for integrating high-resolution multimodality data with EEG. The study investigated the physiologic response of nonconvulsive seizures after subarachnoid hemorrhage. Each minute of EEG was classified after visual inspection by a blinded experienced electroencephalographer as ictal, ictal–interictal continuum, or nonictal. As an exemplar study, note that this step encapsulates two key problems in working with high-resolution data—the data were first acquired then converted, in this case by a human as opposed to computer, into clinical information. This also served as data reduction from 200 Hz to 1-minute resolution. From here, new onset seizures were defined as lasting at least 5 minutes and preceded by 30 minutes without any seizure activity, and then the seizure onset times were integrated with physiologic data. This required a series of SQL queries to automatically identify new onset seizures meeting both criteria and then to link the physiologic data stored in a different database by the defined time window. Physiologic signals were preprocessed through several steps of filtration and missing data were extrapolated. Significance was assessed by constructing a permutation test where investigators resampled by patient and evaluated a Monte Carlo estimate of the significance level.

There are similar strengths and weaknesses of this study to the bedside-to-bench study by Cohen et al (8), discussed previously. The critical point here is to consider them in respect to one's own research questions and capabilities. Like Cohen et al (20), this study was a multidisciplinary effort with investigators from the Department of Neurology, Division of Critical Care Neurology and Comprehensive Epilepsy Center, Department of Neurosurgery, and Department of Biomedical Informatics. Both of these studies required considerable clinical, data management, and analysis expertise. A potential long-term limitation to the Claassen et al (20) study is that this bedside-to-bench study does not have a clear pathway back to the bedside. First, it relies on a human to classify seizures, which may be a limiting factor until ICU seizure detection algorithms improve. Second, a clinical system to send real-time analysis results back to the bedside would need to be developed in order to evaluate these findings. A clinical decision support system (CDSS) is a computer program designed to help clinicians make diagnosis or management decisions (21) and often relies on both patient-specific and knowledge-based information (22). Commercial systems are beginning to address the infrastructure necessary to analyze and deliver results to the bedside in real-time. This is a critical capability for two-way translational research, the importance of which cannot be overstated. It should be planned from the beginning.

LOW-RESOLUTION DATA

Electronic Health Record

Hospitals are spending considerable resources toward electronic health record (EHR) adoption and complying with "meaningful use" standards (23,24). Such systems include electronic prescribing, health information exchange among clinicians and hospitals, and automated reporting of quality performance (23). It is likely that the hospital already has a plan in place to digitize laboratory, clinical exam, intervention, medication, and other tertiary data normally documented on paper charts. All of these data are essential to incorporate into neurophysiologic databases. Again, for epidemiologic and clinical trials acquiring physiologic data from the EHR may be sufficient and the additional effort required to handle high-resolution data can be avoided. It is also unlikely that high-resolution patient monitoring data will be included in EHR systems as these systems are generally not designed to capture and store high resolution physiologic data. Regarding EEG information in the EHR, best case would be documentation in the form of a clinical report for a monitoring period. While nurses do document information from infusion pumps in the EHR, it is well documented that the accuracy is not very good (25–27). There are certain limitations to acquiring data from the EHR that should be recognized.

Ideally one can retrieve these data through a request to a hospital data warehouse group. A data warehouse is a collection of decision-support technologies to enable better and faster decisions (28), and is where lab, imaging, intervention, physiologic, and all other patient databases reside. Traditional data warehouses are set up to bring several different kinds of data (eg, lab and physiologic) together into a unified database to be utilized by clinical support software tools. A data warehouse is a critical component for clinical informatics translational research whereby new uses of patient information can be researched and then brought to the bedside for clinical use through the implementation of a clinical decision support system.

Clinical Data Collection

No matter how much data one is able to acquire from bedside monitors and the EHR, prospective clinical data collection is a vital aspect of both epidemiologic and translational research. You will need to develop a plan on what data to collect, how to collect them, store them in a database, and devise strategies on how to integrate these data with multimodality data. The National Institute of Neurological Disorders and Stroke (NINDS) Common Data Element (CDE) Project has the goal to develop data standards for neurologic research. In addition to having access to tools to help with the creation of paper clinical research forms, collecting common data elements will help facilitate the comparison of results across studies and aggregate information into metadata results (29). This last point is vital for neuromonitoring research since no one center alone is likely to accumulate enough patients to generate definitive results. Prospectively tracking and time-locking clinical complications and secondary events including neurologic, cardiac, and infectious using standard definitions will enable a richer set of research questions to be addressed. This does, however, take more time than simply documenting patient events and treatments as simply a binary yes/no. At the time of this writing, I am not aware of a CDE collection tool being available for this purpose.

Methods to Collect and Store Data

Increasingly metadata-driven browser-based tools are available to collect and store data into a database. REDcap is such a system that was developed by investigators at Vanderbilt University to help support investigator-initiated studies. The software itself is free, but you will need computing resources and expertise to maintain it. There are currently over 680 institutional partners with the REDcap project, and it is possible that someone within your institution is already hosting a REDcap server. Getting set up involves creating an Excel spread sheet that defines your variables and form methods to collect the information. The Excel file is loaded into REDcap, and web forms are automatically created.

REDcap has nice features to extract the collected data into a format for analysis. One word of caution is that, while these standard export features will get data into an analysis program, they will not solve the problem of integrating it with neuromonitoring data. At some point in this process it will be vital to be able to manipulate and combine these data together, likely through a sequence of queries. For example, a database query can identify all neuromonitoring data 24 hours prior to the onset of symptomatic vasospasm and summarize the neuromonitoring data using an algorithm. Some queries can take many hours to run but comparatively to doing this task by hand it is very fast. This processed neuromonitoring data can then be linked to clinical data and exported to an analysis program. The key requirement is that you are able to write queries against the different databases and link them together. System administrators may resist this request, but research with high-resolution physiologic data will be significantly more challenging without this capacity.

Digital Storage of Paper Clinical Research Form (CRF) Data

If you decide to collect data on paper CRFs you will still need to enter these data into a database of some kind. Many investigators choose Microsoft Excel for this purpose; however while its ease of use is appealing as a database it creates more problems than it solves. Perhaps no higher profile example of this is the "error" made by Harvard University investigators Carmen Reinhart and Ken Rogoff. Their research established that once the government debt-to-gross domestic product ratio exceeded 90%, economic growth was likely to become stagnant. Their findings had significant impact on economic policy decisions (30), but unfortunately their findings were erroneous due to simple computational and transcription errors (31) that are far too easy to make in Microsoft Excel.

A spreadsheet is composed of independent cells in which one can insert anything. Data can be intermixed with numbers, letters, and long notes to oneself. Column names can be as long as you want and include spaces and special characters. None of this is conducive to importing your data into an analysis program. Each spreadsheet is separated from the other without any good way to combine data from different sheets. Sorting one column without sorting the rest of your data will ruin your entire dataset in one click.

It is much better to use a relational database such as Microsoft SQL Express, which is free. Even Microsoft Access is problematic because it is difficult to share data across databases, which is important for neuromonitoring research, when your physiologic data will reside separately from your clinical data. Microsoft Access files are also more prone to becoming corrupted than a SQL database. One can think of a SQL table as synonymous to a Microsoft Excel sheet. Different tables are connected to each other by a common study identification number. A view or query is a temporary table freshly created each time it is run. How to combine a subset of data from various tables, or databases for that matter, is not difficult to learn. The ability to query across databases can be leveraged to organize projects by creating a database for each study or manuscript and pulling relevant data from the primary databases. Data entry forms can be created in any web tool that has the ability to connect to a SQL database, for instance REDcap runs on MYSQL which is a variation of Microsoft SQL Express.

SUMMARY

Creating the infrastructure necessary to employ a successful neuromonitoring translational research program is currently feasible and commercial resources are available to help with this process. The key to success is recognizing that there are four challenges to be considered, including: (a) data collection, (b) conversion of raw data into clinical information through analysis, (c) providing clinical information to the bedside in the right format in real time, and (d) integrating this information into clinical workflow. Together these components make up a two-way translational research platform for multimodality monitoring research.

REFERENCES

1. Wartenberg KE, Schmidt JM, Mayer SA. Multimodality monitoring in neurocritical care. *Crit Care Clin*. 2007;23:507–538.
2. Mayberg MR, Okada T, Bark DH. Morphologic changes in cerebral arteries after subarachnoid hemorrhage. *Neurosurg Clin N Am*. 1990;1:417–432.
3. Kononenko I, Kukar M. *Machine learning and data mining: Introduction to principles and algorithms*. Horwood Pub Ltd; 2007.
4. The NIH Common Fund. Re-engineering the Clinical Research Enterprise. 2009. http://nihroadmap.nih.gov/clinicalresearch/overview-translational.asp. Accessed July 10, 2013.
5. Marincola FM. Translational medicine: A two way road. *J Transl Med*. 2003;1:1.
6. Jacono FJ, De Georgia MA, Wilson CG, et al. Data acquisition and complex systems analysis in critical care: Developing the intensive care unit of the future. *Journal of Healthcare Engineering*. 2010;1:337–355.
7. Buchman TG. Novel representation of physiologic states during critical illness and recovery. *Crit Care*. 2010;14:127.
8. Cohen MJ, Grossman AD, Morabito D, et al. Identification of complex metabolic states in critically injured patients using bioinformatic cluster analysis. *Crit Care*. 2010;14:R10.

9. Bardt TF, Unterberg AW, Hartl R, et al. Monitoring of brain tissue PO_2 in traumatic brain injury: Effect of cerebral hypoxia on outcome. *Acta Neurochir Suppl.* 1998;71:153–156.

10. Maloney-Wilensky E, Le Roux P. The physiology behind direct brain oxygen monitors and practical aspects of their use. *Childs Nerv Syst.* 2010;26:419-430.

11. Lake DE, Richman JS, Griffin MP, et al. Sample entropy analysis of neonatal heart rate variability. *Am J Physiol Regul Integr Comp Physiol.* 2002;283:R789–797.

12. Moorman JR, Lake DE, Griffin MP. Heart rate characteristics monitoring for neonatal sepsis. *Biomedical Engineering, IEEE Transactions on.* 2006;53:126–132.

13. Moorman JR, Carlo WA, Kattwinkel J, et al. Mortality reduction by heart rate characteristic monitoring in very low birth weight neonates: A randomized trial. *The Journal of pediatrics.* 2011.

14. Steiner LA, Czosnyka M, Piechnik SK, et al. Continuous monitoring of cerebrovascular pressure reactivity allows determination of optimal cerebral perfusion pressure in patients with traumatic brain injury. *Crit Care Med.* 2002;30:733–738.

15. Kull L, Emerson R. Continuous eeg monitoring in the intensive care unit: Technical and staffing considerations. *Journal of Clinical Neurophysiology.* 2005;22:107–118.

16. Chelico J, PhD A, Wajngurt D. Architectural design of a data warehouse to support operational and analytical queries across disparate clinical databases. 2007:901.

17. Martich G, Waldmann C, Imhoff M. Clinical informatics in critical care. *Journal of Intensive Care Medicine.* 2004;19:154.

18. Chou D, Sengupta S. *Infrastructure and security.* Burlington, MA: Academic Press; 2008.

19. Kull LL, Emerson RG. Continuous eeg monitoring in the intensive care unit: Technical and staffing considerations. *J Clin Neurophysiol.* 2005;22:107–118.

20. Claassen J, Perotte A, Albers D, et al. Nonconvulsive seizures after subarachnoid hemorrhage: Multimodal detection and outcomes. *Ann Neurol.* 2013.

21. Musen M, Shahar Y, Shortliffe E. Clinical decision-support systems. *Biomedical Informatics.* 2006:698–736.

22. Hersh W. Medical informatics: Improving health care through information. *Jama.* 2002;288:1955.

23. Jha A. Meaningful use of electronic health records. *JAMA: The Journal of the American Medical Association.* 2010;304:1709.

24. Jha A, DesRoches C, Kralovec P, et al. A progress report on electronic health records in us hospitals. *Health Affairs.* 2010;29:1951.

25. Sapo M, Wu S, Asgari S, et al. A comparison of vital signs charted by nurses with automated acquired values using waveform quality indices. *Journal of Clinical Monitoring and Computing.* 2009;23:263–271.

26. Vawdrey D, Gardner R, Evans R, et al. Assessing data quality in manual entry of ventilator settings. *J Am Med Inform Assoc.* 2007;14:295–303.

27. Dalto JD, Johnson KV, Gardner RM, et al. Medical information bus usage for automated iv pump data acquisition: Evaluation of usage patterns. *Int J Clin Monit Comput.* 1997;14:151–154.

28. Chaudhuri S, Dayal U. An overview of data warehousing and olap technology. *ACM Sigmod record.* 1997;26:65–74.

29. NINDS common data element project. 2013.

30. Summers L. Lessons can be learned from Reinhart-Rogoff error. *The Washington Post.* May 5, 2013.

31. Baker, Dean. How much unemployment was caused by Reinhart and Rogoff's arithmetic mistake? April 16, 2013. Available at http://www.cepr.net/index.php/blogs/beat-the-press/how-much-unemployment-was-caused-by-reinhart-and-rogoffs-arithmetic-mistake

Nursing: The Essential Piece to Successful Neuromonitoring

Tess Slazinski, RN, MN, CCRN, CNRN, CCNS

INTRODUCTION

Neurocritical care units were created for the purpose of enhancing the capacity for patient monitoring and provision of neuro-specific care. While these goals require the effort and collaboration of various team members, the involvement of the neurocritical care nurse is perhaps most central and essential to the achievement of this objective. By serial performance of a detailed neurologic exam with unprecedented expertise, the neurocritical care nurse was the first "neuromonitor." Throughout the years, advances in biomedical technology have created an array of mechanical neuromonitors capable of identifying structural and physiologic changes that precede patient deterioration. The implementation, use, and trouble shooting of these neuromonitors has chiefly depended upon the knowledge and proficiency of both neurocritical care and advanced practice nurses (APNs). This chapter focuses upon strategies for successful training of the neurocritical care nurse and the role of the nurse in neuromonitoring. The responsibility of the APN in developing a successful neuromonitoring unit is also addressed.

The American Association of Neurosurgical Nurses (AANN) was founded in 1968 in affiliation with the American Association of Neurological Surgeons (AANS). The AANN was founded to recognize the common needs of nurses caring for neuroscience patients and to provide a forum for these nurses to share concerns. The American Nurses Association (ANA) defines specialization as "involving a focus on nursing practice in a specific area, identified from within the whole field of professional nursing. ANA and specialty nursing organizations delineate the components of professional nursing practice that are essential for any particular specialty" (1). The AANN has evolved into a separate entity, entitled the American Association of Neuroscience Nurses, to encompass both neurological and neurosurgical patient populations. The organization has special focus groups to appreciate the various subspecialties within neuroscience nursing. In addition, the Neurocritical Care Society (NCS) has realized the importance of the neuroscience intensive care unit (ICU) nurses by supporting MD/RN collaborative practice (eg, dual workshop presentations and clinical practice guidelines authorship).

NEUROSCIENCE INTENSIVE CARE UNIT NURSING PERSONNEL

Hospitals that have achieved Comprehensive Stroke Center (CSC) status appreciate the training that is necessary for neuroscience ICU nurses. The CSC guidelines have the highest hourly education requirement for nurses in the neuroscience ICU setting. In addition, a noticeable achievement in the CSC guidelines is the recognition of contributions made by APNs. The guidelines state that a nurse practitioner (NP) or clinical nurse specialist (CNS) needs to author and oversee the educational content (2). The content expertise is in the following areas: treatment of increased intracranial pressure monitoring, hemodynamic monitoring, ventilator management, external ventricular devices management, ischemic and hemorrhagic stroke, hypothermia management, post t-PA administration care, and so forth (2). Although this is not an exhaustive list of all the items neuroscience ICU nurses should have in their armamentarium, its existence represents subspecialty nursing progress.

APNs consist of nurse practitioners and clinical nurse specialists. APNs are nurses who are master's or doctorally prepared. Acute care nurse practitioners (ACNPs) scope of practice includes diagnosis and treatment of complex acute and chronic medical problems, prescriptive authority, and the ability to perform procedures according to training in the emergency department or ICU settings. The ACNP, with the proper ICU training, provides high quality, cost-effective patient care (3).

The clinical nurse specialist (CNS) practices within multiple spheres of influence, a feature which is both essential and unique to the role. The CNS is a clinical expert who manages complex and vulnerable patients; a researcher and educator charged with moving multidisciplinary practice forward; and a facilitator of change and innovation within a system to enhance quality and outcomes. The CNS's advanced education includes advanced clinical skills, research analysis and implementation, and systems-level project planning. In addition, the CNS translates evidence-based practice to the bedside nurse (3).

Competent bedside nurses are essential to the neuroscience ICU. Although individual nursing schools have different training programs, they do not prepare the new graduate nurse for sub specialty nursing (4). Hospitals may also have varying schools of thought about how to assess competencies for bedside nurses, but the ANA and The Joint Commission have specific recommendations for competency-based orientation programs. These programs need to include tools that capture objective and subjective data, while ensuring patient safety (5). In addition, these competency tools need to be part of a dynamic, ongoing educational process (5). The challenge for CNSs is how to present the necessary information in new employee orientation in order to achieve the greatest amount of learning (6). This challenge is compounded by the nursing shortage (6). Due to the nursing shortage, retention and recruitment for the ICU is a major priority for many hospitals. The essential components to recruitment and retention are proper hiring and orientation.

HIRING

The CNS, as part of nursing leadership, is trained to ask the strategic clinical questions (7) in new employee interviews and should be included in the interview process. These interviews may be conducted together or separately from the manager interview. It is rare to find experienced neuro-ICU nurses. In the era of cost containment, an experienced non-neuro ICU nurse can be trained to a new facility within a shorter period of time (6).

The following questions are examples used for experienced ICU nurse interviews at a large, teaching hospital:

- What two ECG leads do we monitor from at the bedside?
- What are the troubleshooting strategies nurses utilize when the patient has an over dampened arterial line waveform?
- What are the nursing management components to the care of a patient with a chest tube?
- What are common high-pressure ventilator alarms?
- Have you cared for patients with external ventricular drains (EVDs)?
- Tell us about a patient situation in which you noticed a change in the patient's physiologic parameters and made a difference in the patient's outcome?

The preceding questions assist units in determining which candidates have worked with varying types of equipment and possess critical thinking skills. If a new graduate or new to specialty (non-ICU, step-down unit) nurses are interviewed, the questions are focused on basic nursing assessment and step-down unit experience:

- What two ECG leads do we monitor from at the bedside?
- What is the normal hourly urine output?
- Where do we place the stethoscope to listen for S1 and S2?
- What are abnormal breath sounds?
- Have you cared for patients with a lumbar drain?

NEUROSCIENCE ICU TRAINING (ORIENTATION)

The key to any successful neuroscience ICU program is support by the entire team (8). Team members who provide support by recognizing the important of nursing training include: neurointensivists, neurosurgeons, neurologists, acute care nurse practitioners (ACNP), pharmacists, therapists, and social workers. In addition, nursing directors and managers oversee the financial support that is vital to the success of any neuroscience ICU program.

Critical care orientation programs need to include lectures, visual cues, and tactile experiences (9,10). Embedded within this curriculum is unit-specific content. It is the APN's responsibility to develop a neuroscience ICU nursing core curriculum based on the unit's patient population. Not all neuroscience ICUs have the same patient populations. For example, some units may have more traumatic brain injury (TBI) patients versus other units that have more aneurysmal subarachnoid hemorrhage (aSAH) patients. The focus of the curriculum content is determined by number of unit admissions and easily tracked by ICD-10 codes. The common patient populations admitted into a neuro-science ICU are the following: hemorrhagic stroke, ischemic stroke, TBI, status epilepti-cus, cerebral neoplasms, infectious central nervous system diseases, and complex spine surgery. Each new neuroscience ICU nurse should receive the same clinical content. An example of content delineation is illustrated in Table 11.1. Each class should provide content that builds from one class to the next. At the course completion, each participant needs to complete written and oral examinations. The written examination should be a

TABLE 11.1 Neuroscience Nursing Core Curriculum

CONTENT TITLE	DESCRIPTION	HOURS
1. Correlative brain anatomy and neurologic assessment	The neuroanatomy course provides a broad overview of the structure and function of the central nervous system, with a principal focus on issues relevant to the bedside neuroscience ICU nurse. The class consists of lecture, hands-on with brain models and anatomical brain slices. The neurologic examination includes: mental status, cranial nerves, motor, sensory, and the cerebellum as it relates to the alert and nonalert patients.	4
2. Ischemic and hemorrhagic stroke	The ischemic and hemorrhagic stroke content will be presented in lecture format. The lecture will provide information about the causes, categories, medical treatment, and nursing management for both types of stroke.	2
3. Traumatic brain injury	The TBI content explores the different mechanism of injuries, categories of traumatic hemorrhages, medical diagnosis, and nursing management.	1
4. Intracranial pressure monitoring (ICP)	The ICP course describes the types of brain herniation, and nursing maneuvers to reduce increased ICP. The ICP devices includes fiberoptic and external ventricular drain setup via simulation.	2
5. Cerebral neoplasms	The cerebral neoplasm lecture provides the learner with knowledge about types, the diagnosis, surgical management, and nursing management for patients with brain tumors.	1
6. Spinal cord anatomy	The spinal cord anatomy content describes the bony anatomy, spinal cord anatomy, and key pathways.	1
7. Spinal cord injury (SCI)	The SCI lecture includes different mechanisms of injury, spinal cord syndromes, and nursing management.	30 minutes
8. Complex spine surgery	The complex spine surgery lecture defines different surgical approaches and fixation hardware, and nursing management.	30 minutes

multiple-choice test, written in the style of the board examinations (ie, CCRN, CNRN, SCRN). The oral examination should consist of performing the neurologic assessment.

ORIENTATION SPECIFIC TO MULTIMODAL NEUROMONITORING

Many nursing articles exist regarding multimodal neuromonitoring and nursing interventions to decrease intracranial pressure (11–21). These articles provide nurses with information about pathophysiology, advanced equipment, and data interpretation. This information may be included in orientation curricula but cannot provide information about psychomotor skills and real-time bedside interpretation. Very few resources exist regarding the specific educational requirements for nurses who are new to the neuroscience ICU setting.

Clinical nurse specialists and educators understand that each piece of equipment requires a policy and procedure and a competency checklist. In addition to CNSs and educators possessing knowledge about evidence-based clinical practice guidelines and procedure manuals, new staff should be familiar with these resources. The *AACN Procedure Manual* (22–25) has chapters that are dedicated to multimodal neuromonitoring. The *AANN Clinical Practice Guidelines* (CPG; 26) on external ventricular drains (EVDs) and lumbar drainage devices (LDDs) provides the bedside nurse with a step-by-step procedure for priming the devices, which no other published material contains. Is it enough for a new staff nurse to read a policy and procedure without simulation? Allowing individuals with minimal training to operate complex equipment can be hazardous for patients because of the possibility of operator error (27). The following are examples of the key components for a successful multimodal neuromonitoring training program: preceptor orientation, simulation training, and annual competencies.

Nursing preceptors are an important part of nursing orientation and need to receive proper training prior to training new staff. The preceptors should attend a hospital preceptor class and advanced training on equipment, so they can field questions in the absence of the CNS. In addition, the preceptors need to describe the implications and advantages of multimodal neuromonitoring. Multimodal neuromonitoring involves appreciation of the following (27):

■ Monitoring several variables simultaneously will provide information on different aspects of brain physiology

■ Patients will require more intense nursing care and several interventions performed at once

■ Learning new patient management strategies

■ Technical proficiency of new equipment

An example of advanced training content is listed in Table 11.2. The preceptor's ability to answer questions about equipment or patient management, gives the autonomy that is necessary for job satisfaction and retention (6,8).

Simulation training involves equipment assembly and setup. Each new employee needs to locate the necessary equipment and demonstrate how to set it up. For example, the EVD

TABLE 11.2 Advanced Neuromonitoring Content

CONTENT TITLE	DESCRIPTION	HOURS
1. Nursing management for the patient with increased intracranial pressure (ICP)	The lecture provides nurses with a review of the etiology of increased ICP, types of ICP monitoring, advanced neuromonitoring devices, and nursing maneuvers to decrease ICP.	1
2. Brain tissue oxygen monitoring (PbtO$_2$)	The lecture provides nurses with information about cerebral oxygen supply and demand, and brain tissue oxygen and temperature monitoring devices. In addition, each nurse is provided optimal time to set up the equipment in simulation.	1

supplies should be on a line cart or centrally located on the unit. The flushless transducer needs to be located in an area separate from flush transducers. In addition, the advanced neuromonitoring (ie, SjVO$_2$, PbtO$_2$, and microdialysis) equipment should be in a designated, secure location. Often, the unit champion is the CNS, who makes herself or himself available to assist with all of these procedures until the staff are comfortable with equipment assembly and setup. After multiple insertions of advanced neuromonitoring products has occurred, other unit champions can be added. Each staff member is required to complete a competency checklist for all new products. Examples of competency checklists are listed in the appendices.

The final component of multimodal neuromonitoring is ongoing assessment of competencies. Ongoing competencies can be assessed in an annual skills day format, which is usually a mandatory requirement for every staff member. Skills days can be conducted 1:1 or in small groups. The CNS often checks off the unit experts, who then check off the less experienced staff. This type of unit participation is important for promoting teamwork. In addition to the psychomotor skills, each staff member is required to state the indications, troubleshooting, and nursing management for each piece of equipment.

The NPs and CNSs are in opportune leadership positions to assess ongoing skill acquisition. While performing daily rounds, they may ascertain whether or not the bedside nurses understand the patient diagnosis and plan of care. Teaching opportunities arise on a daily basis with acutely ill neuroscience patients, and it is important for bedside nurses to embrace the challenge of the answering clinical questions.

Examples of pertinent clinical questions are the following:

■ What is diffuse axonal injury?

■ Where is a fiberoptic catheter sitting inside the brain?

■ What are the normal components of the ICP waveform?

■ Which component of the ICP waveform demonstrates decreased compliance?

■ What is a normal PbtO$_2$?

■ What are factors that increase brain tissue oxygen demand?

■ What are factors that decrease brain tissue oxygen supply?

■ Why is it important to monitor brain temperature?

■ How does burst suppression appear on the continuous EEG monitor?

CONCLUSION

A neuroscience ICU nurse needs to receive the proper clinical content and simulation training in order to provide competent, safe patient care. The clinical content must be population driven and include several teaching modalities. Teaching modalities include lecture, interactive case study presentations, and equipment assembly and setup.

Multimodal neuromonitoring provides the bedside nurse with a plethora of data to interpret. A team approach is required to collect, analyze, and treat the patient accordingly. Continuous follow-up at the bedside is needed to ensure understanding of this very complex, challenging patient population. Future research is needed in the field of neuroscience ICU nursing education to determine cost effectiveness and patient outcomes.

REFERENCES

1. American Nurses' Association. 2008. Professional role competence (position paper). Retrieved from http.//www.nursingworld.org/NursingPractice.
2. The Joint Commission. Recommendations for comprehensive stroke center. 2011.
3. Bauman JJ, Rinaldo L. Nurse practitioner or clinical nurse specialist: Which do you need? *Currents*, 2013;8(2):16.
4. Square N. Modeling clinical applications in intensive care settings for nursing orientation. *Advances in Neonatal Care*, 2010;10(6):325–329.
5. Wolfensperger-Bashford C, Shaffer B, Young C. Assessment of clinical judgment in nursing orientation. *Journal of Nurses in Staff Development*, 2012;28(2):62–65.
6. Thomason T. ICU nursing orientation and post orientation practices. *Critical Care Nursing Quarterly*. 2006;29(3):237–245.
7. Jarouse L. Best practices for recruitment and retention. *Hospitals & Health Networks*. Accessed June 28, 2013.
8. Brakovich B, Boham E. Solving the retention puzzle: Let's begin with nursing Orientation. *Nurse Leader*, 2012, 50–61.
9. Culley T, Babbie A, Clancey J., et al. Nursing U: A new concept for nursing orientation. *Nursing Management*, March 2012, 45–47.
10. Dunbar K, Radsliff E. Integrating simulation into hospital nursing orientation. Presentation abstracts from 2012 INACSL conference. *Clinical simulation in nursing*, 2012;8(8):e401.
11. Littlejohns L, Bader MK, March K. Brain tissue oxygen monitoring in severe brain injury, I: Research and usefulness in critical care. *Critical Care Nurse*, 2003;23:17–25.
12. Bader MK, Littlejohns L, March K. Brain tissue oxygen monitoring in severe brain injury, II: Implications for critical care teams and case study. *Critical Care Nurse*, 2003;23:29–44.
13. Wilensky EM, Bloom S, Leicter D., et al. Brain tissue oxygen practice guidelines using the LICOX CMP monitoring system. *Journal of Neuroscience Nursing*, 2005;37:278–288.
14. Bader MK. Gizmos and gadgets for the neuroscience intensive care unit. *Journal of Neuroscience Nursing*, 2006;38(4):248–260.
15. Rauen CA, Chulay M, Bridges E., et al. Seven evidence-based practice habits: Putting some sacred cows out to pasture. *Critical Care Nurse*, 2008;28:98–123.
16. Rupich K. The use of hypothermia as a treatment for traumatic brain injury. *Journal of Neuroscience Nursing*, 2009;41(3):159–167.
17. Prescuitti MJ, Schmidt M, Alexander S. Neuromonitoring in intensive care: Focus on microdialysis and its nursing implications. *Journal of Neuroscience Nursing*, 2009;41(3):131–139.
18. Cecil S, Chen PM, Calloway S., et al. Traumatic brain injury: Advanced multimodal neuromonitoring from theory to clinical practice. *Critical Care Nurse*, 2010;31(2):25–36.

19. Prescuitti M, Bader MK, Hepburn M. Shivering management during therapeutic temperature modulation: Nurses' perspective. *Critical Care Nurse*, 2012;32:33–42.

20. Seiler E, Fields J, Peach E., et al. The effectiveness of a staff education program on the use of continuous EEG with patients in neuroscience intensive care units. *Journal of Neuroscience Nursing*, 2012;44(2):E1–E5.

21. McNett MM, Olson D. Evidence to guide nursing interventions for critically ill neurologically impaired patients with ICP monitoring. *Journal of Neuroscience Nursing*, 2013;45(1):120–123.

22. Wilensky EM, Bloom SA, Stiefel MF. Brain tissue oxygen monitoring: Insertion (assist), care, and troubleshooting. In Blissett, P. (Section Ed.). *AACN Procedure Manual for Critical Care Nurses* (6th ed). St. Louis, MO: Elsevier Sanders, 2011:792–801.

23. Slazinski, T. Intracranial bolt and fiberoptic catheter insertion (assist), intracranial pressure monitoring, care, troubleshooting, and removal. In Blissett, P. (Section Ed.). *AACN Procedure Manual for Critical Care Nurses* (6th ed., 802-808). St. Louis, MO: Elsevier Saunders, 2011;802–808.

24. Slazinski, T. Combination intraventricular/fiberoptic catheter insertion (assist), monitoring, nursing care, troubleshooting, and removal. In Blissett, P. (Section Ed.). *AACN Procedure Manual for Critical Care Nurses* (6th ed). St. Louis, MO: Elsevier Saunders, 2011;809–815.

25. Slazinski, T. Jugular venous oxygen saturation monitoring: insertion (assist), patient care, troubleshooting, and removal. In Blissett, P. (Section Ed.). *AACN Procedure Manual for Critical Care Nurses* (6th ed.). St. Louis, MO: Elsevier Saunders, 2011;816–825.

26. Thompson, H. & Slazinski, T. (Eds.). Care of the patient undergoing intracranial pressure monitoring/EVD/LDD. In *AANN Clinical Practice Guideline*. Glenview, IL: AANN, 2011.

27. Keow LK, Dip Adv, Ng Ivan. The implications of multimodal neuromonitoring for nursing. *Singapore Nursing Journal*. 2005;32(4):5–11.

APPENDIX A

External Ventricular Drainage (EVD)

Name:_____Title:_____Unit:_____

VALIDATOR'S INITIALS	SKILL	EVALUATION METHOD
	Assemble the following equipment:	
	1) Cranial access kit	DO, SIM
	2) Ventricular catheter	
	3) Drainage collection device	
	4) Transducer (*flushless*)	
	Assemble the drainage collection device:	
	1) Attach external transducer (*flushless*)	DO, SIM
	2) Prime tubing with *preservative free* normal saline	
	Drainage collection device maintenance:	
	1) Describe the anatomical landmark for zero reference level and demonstrate how to level transducer.	DO, SIM
	2) Describe where to place the pressure level (graduated burette).	
	3) Demonstrate how to zero to atmosphere.	
	4) Demonstrate how to change the collection bag (mask and gloves).	
	5) Describe how often CSF drainage is measured.	
	6) Demonstrate checking EVD for patency.	
	Demonstrate use of cables to patient side:	
	1) Attach transducer cable to the bedside monitor.	DO, SIM
	2) Demonstrate how to zero the transducer and describe how often transducer needs to be re-zeroed.	
	Use of alarms:	
	1) Set bedside alarms—state normal values.	DO, SIM
	Troubleshooting: most common problems listed:	
	1) Not draining:	DO, SIM
	—Graduated burette set too high	
	—Tubing clotted off	
	—Ventricles collapsed	
	—Clamps in "off" position	

VALIDATOR'S INITIALS	SKILL	EVALUATION METHOD
	2) Dampened waveform: —Air across transducer —Pressure transducer set too low	DO, SIM
	3) Disconnection: —Clamp end of ventricular catheter or EVD tubing with sterile 4 X 4 and hemostat —Setup new EVD drainage system —Call house officer	DO, SIM

Technique Standard Met:	☐ Yes ☐ No
Demonstration Date:	
Validator's Name:	
Validator's Signature:	

Evaluation Method:

DO = Directly observed individual performing critical skill

SIM = Individual simulated performing critical skill

CA = A chart audit reflected performance of skill

Verbal = Cognitive testing reflects theoretical basis of critical skill

APPENDIX B

Fiberoptic catheter

Name:_____Title:_____Unit:_____

VALIDATOR'S SIGNATURE	SKILL	EVALUATION METHOD
	Assemble necessary equipment for fiberoptic catheter placement:	
	1. Cranial access kit (contains drill)	DO, SIM
	2. Fiberoptic catheter (MRI safety versus compatibility)	
	a. ICP only	
	b. Licox (ICP, $PbtO_2$, and temperature)	
	3. Camino MPM monitor	
	Assemble the following rear panel cables:	
	1. Cable to bedside and importance of knowing the bedside monitor configuration	DO, SIM
	2. Power cord—needs to be charged when not in use; articulates length of battery life	
	3. Plug in to temperature and parenchymal ports	
	4. Troubleshooting guide in pocket of rear panel	
	Demonstrate use of front panel buttons:	
	1. "Scale" for adjusting to meet the needs of dampened waveform, elevated ICP or negative value	DO, SIM
	2. "Synchronize " to bedside monitor	
	3. "Trend" (data)	
	Use of alarms:	
	1. Setting bedside ICP alarm/states normal values	DO, SIM
	2. Setting bedside CPP alarm/states normal values	
	3. Disabling MPM alarms and pausing alarm—how long does it stay silenced	

VALIDATOR'S SIGNATURE	SKILL	EVALUATION METHOD
	Troubleshooting: Most common problems listed	
	1. Negative number: a. Hemovac or Jackson pratt next to the catheter? b. Large dose of Mannitol after OR? c. Patient has a basilar skull fracture?	DO, SIM
	2. Number too high: a. White compression cap at the bolt is anchored too tight? b. Catheter not brought back 1 mm during insertion?	DO, SIM

Technique Standard Met:	☐ Yes	☐ No
Demonstration Date:		
Validator's Name:		
Validator's Signature:		

Evaluation Method:

DO = Directly observed individual performing critical skill

SIM = Individual simulated performing critical skill

CA = A chart audit reflected performance of skill

Verbal = Cognitive testing reflects theoretical basis of critical skill

APPENDIX C

Brain Tissue Oxygen Monitor (Licox™)

Name:_____Title:_____Unit:_____

VALIDATOR'S INITIALS	SKILL	EVALUATION METHOD
	Assemble/prepare the following equipment:	
	1) Check Licox™ CMP monitor to ensure all cables are connected.	DO, SIM
	2) Prepare for a sterile procedure.	
	3) Assist the neurosurgeon or neurointensivist with placement of bolt introducer, brain tissue oxygen and temperature probes, and tissue ICP probes.	
	4) Ensure power cord is connected at rear of the monitor.	
	5) Ensure blue oxygen cable and green temperature cable or PMO combination catheter is connected on the front panel.	DO, SIM
	6) Turn the monitor on (switch on back of machine).	
	7) Insert the smart card from the oxygen probe introducer package into the slot on the front panel until it snaps into position.	DO, SIM
	8) Connect the PMO catheter to the PMO connector (combined oxygen and temperature probes) on monitor.	
	9) Wait approximately 20–30 minutes to begin recording of $PbtO_2$ values.	
	10) Disconnect the Licox™ probes at the patient end in the event transport to the CT scanner, MRI or operating room is needed.	
	Knows that brain tissue oxygen monitor probe and bolt must be removed prior to MRI study.	
	Maintenance:	
	1) Assess status of insertion site.	DO, SIM
	2) Change dressing as necessary.	
	3) Monitor, document, and report delayed drainage from site.	DO, SIM
	4) Report any bleeding, excessive drainage or any signs of infection.	DO, SIM
	5) Refers to Licox™ CMP brain oxygen monitoring system operations manual for further information on alarms, trouble shooting, and other information.	DO, SIM
	6) Assess bolt mechanism hourly to verify bolt and catheter connectivity.	DO, SIM
	7) Inspect bolt insertion site each shift and reports any redness, purulence, skin breakdown, leakage, or instability.	DO, SIM

Technique Standard Met:	☐ Yes ☐ No
Demonstration Date:	
Validator's Name:	
Validator's Signature:	

Evaluation Method:

DO = Directly observed individual performing critical skill

SIM = Individual simulated performing critical skill

CA = A chart audit reflected performance of skill

Verbal = Cognitive testing reflects theoretical basis of critical skill

Multimodal Monitoring: Challenges in Implementation and Clinical Utilization

Chad M. Miller, MD

INTRODUCTION

The accumulation of data demonstrating the worth of various neuromonitors in identifying cerebral injury, assisting in prognosis, and personalizing provision of care would portend that neuromonitoring implementation is widespread and utilization has become standard of care (1,2). In fact, comprehensive neuromonitoring is employed less often than opportunity would allow. Historically, invasive neuromonitoring has flourished in centers where individuals have supported and championed its use, but in those centers without dedicated neurocritical care units, its popularity has lagged. Several barriers and challenges to multimodal monitoring (MMM) implementation limit the potential impact of these technologies. This chapter focuses on the current benefits, misunderstandings, limitations, and unjustified expectations surrounding MMM. The chapter will also suggest the measures that are essential in addressing each of these concerns.

OUTCOMES DATA

MMM excels at identification of secondary brain injury that is often not apparent without its use. The vast majority of literature addressing MMM can be classified as descriptive observational research that equates monitor thresholds to outcome and survival (3). Despite this evidence, perhaps the most common critique of MMM is the lack of proven efficacy of monitor driven treatment paradigms. In some circumstances, there remains uncertainty regarding those monitoring thresholds most highly correlated with outcome, or furthermore, if the monitors are detecting physiologic processes that are therapeutically modifiable. This criticism is not new or unique to newer-generation neuromonitoring devices. For years, controversy has surrounded pulmonary artery catheters and their use in understanding complex hemodynamic physiology (4). Whether resulting from improper use, misunderstandings of the extrapolation of volume data from pressure recordings, or simply the frustration of unsatisfactory results, this technology has been slowly phased out of routine use in the critical care unit. More traditional neuromonitoring devices initially escaped similar criticism, but their role in delivering improved outcomes is just now being evaluated after decades of unquestioned utilization. Few would argue the value of intracranial pressure (ICP) monitoring for use in guiding care of patients with intracranial hypertension. However, the clinical benefits of ICP monitoring are unproven and recent studies have begun to question the standard thresholds adopted in treatment guidelines, as well as the validity of treatment protocols based solely upon ICP derived targets (5).

To what expectations should MMM be judged? It is clear the neuromonitors excel at identification of occult brain injury and tissue at risk and their detection has greater sensitivity than basic monitoring methods such as neurologic exams and radiologic imaging (6). Is lack of demonstrated improved outcomes clearly a monitor failure, or rather a consequence of ineffective therapies or reactive and late therapeutic intervention? Monitors are most fairly judged by their capacity to perform their intended function: identification of risk for secondary brain injury. While it is fair to desire that MMM eventually become better integrated into therapeutic protocols that improve clinical outcomes, this endpoint reflects much more than the capability of the monitor. The onus is on the innovation of the neurocritical care community to improve upon the ways of utilizing current neuromonitoring. This will invariably require a refined understanding of MMM treatment thresholds, timeliness of intervention, determination of effective treatments, and appreciation of the complementary value of various monitoring devices. While many of these aims require future development, our current knowledge of the pathophysiology of brain injury justifies the individualization of care afforded by MMM.

COMMITMENT TO MULTIMODAL MONITORING: ASSEMBLING THE MULTIDISCIPLINARY TEAM

MMM requires commitment to the process. The neurocritical care team is commonly composed of surgeons, intensivists, nurses, advanced practice nurses, pharmacists, residents, and trainees, each with disparate experience and varying understanding of the importance of secondary injury and the value and role of neuromonitoring. Since implementation of invasive MMM is not easy and probe placement carries some risk to the patient, there is a natural tendency for some physicians to favor conservative neurocritical care management without the use of MMM. However, general conservative treatment protocols fail to address variability in disease course and result in an unacceptable rate of delayed morbidity and mortality. The quest to recognize and address these opportunities is the common rallying point of the MMM team.

A functional MMM program requires a coordinated effort and belief in neuromonitoring (Table 12.1). At many institutions, invasive monitors are placed exclusively by neurosurgeons. Many of these colleagues may not have been trained at an institution that utilized MMM or have personal experience analyzing MMM data. Nonetheless, their role in the timely placement of these monitors is indispensable to the monitoring program. A substantial amount of trust is required for a surgeon to accept the risk of implanting a monitor in his or her patient and subsequently allowing an intensivist to use this information to

TABLE 12.1 Required Fundamentals for Successful Neuromonitoring

Dedicated team of physicians and nurses

Well-specified monitoring indications and protocols

Reasonable expectations for value of monitoring data

Display systems that integrate and allow appropriate scale and comparison of data

Real-time analysis of data to guide therapeutic adjustments

manage the patient in a manner with which the surgeon may not be familiar. Likewise, the nurse and intensivist must be devoted to the value of neuromonitoring to embrace the work of bedside monitoring management and responsive data analysis.

A lapse in dedication of the multidisciplinary chain can result in a lost monitoring opportunity. For many teams, the common belief that justifies and drives the MMM effort is recognition that standard care without MMM routinely fails to identify occult brain injury and prevent permanent disability caused by secondary processes (6). A clearly established protocol to guide patient eligibility and timing for MMM helps to ease concerns among team members regarding the appropriateness and institutional standardization of monitoring.

MULTIMODAL MONITORING AND CLINICAL GUIDELINES

In an era where evidence-based practice is heralded, it is surprising that so few clinical scenarios carry evidence-based solutions. Consequently, many practitioners look to expert opinion from consensus guidelines to direct their management options. International and societal guidelines have been largely silent regarding the role of MMM in management of critical brain disease. The most recent Brain Trauma Foundation Severe TBI, American Heart Association/American Stroke Association (AHA/ASA) Intracerebral Hemorrhage, and AHA/ASA Aneurysmal Subarachnoid Hemorrhage Guidelines provide minimal to no direction regarding the use of multimodal monitoring in impaired and comatose patients (7–9). As a result, there is marked variability among the types, timing, and combinations of neuromonitors used in protocols.

Some of these deficiencies will be addressed with 2014 publication of neuromonitoring guidelines from the International Consensus Conference on Multimodality Monitoring. These guidelines will aim to summarize the current literature in an evidence-based format, recommend monitoring platforms for a multitude of clinical conditions, and establish standardization for monitoring techniques. A comprehensive look at the current state of MMM monitoring is likely to identify deficiencies in our knowledge of monitoring and shape the future of MMM research.

LEARNING TO READ THE TEA LEAVES

Data analysis can be challenging in MMM. Whereas some monitoring output, such as regional cerebral blood flow expressed as cc/100 g/min, has intuitive meaning, other monitors provide data in less clear and familiar terms. Transcranial Doppler ultrasonography estimates blood flow through red blood cell velocity. The expression of brain oxygen delivery by partial pressure of oxygen contradicts our fundamental understanding of oxygen-carrying capacity. The presentation of continuous EEG (cEEG) data in raw form eludes detailed quantitative description. Equally perplexing is the great physiologic variability of many MMM parameters, and the inconsistent use of normal thresholds (1). Is there a universal microdialysis glutamate concentration that should justify clinical concern? Should a lactate:pyruvate ratio (LPR) greater than 25 or 50 cause alarm? Are there instances where these findings are not indicative of ischemic risk? Is a $PbtO_2$ threshold of 15 or 20 mmHg more appropriate? For many monitoring devices, there is a notion that intra-patient trends may be more revealing than absolute values. Real-time analysis that accounts for these considerations is much more difficult to implement and automate.

The complexity of analysis is being resolved through standardization of thresholds and treatment paradigms. Data sharing, research consortia, and collective experience have paved the way for greater consistency in management among institutions.

MULTIMODAL MONITORING: WORTH THE EFFORT

MMM is difficult to do. The technologies can be expensive and physically invasive. Consequently, implementation of MMM must be justified to administrators watching the budget as well as those with less experience regarding its capabilities and value. Nursing staffs and superusers must be on hand at all hours to troubleshoot monitor complications. Many of the neuromonitoring devices are unfamiliar to general critical care nurses and require bedside adjustments from someone who has greater than a novice's knowledge of the technique. To justify the process clinically, the pace of data analysis must mirror the perpetual time course of physiological change. Many neurocritical care units are cross-covered by inexperienced house staff at night, and the complexity of interraled physiological variables require back up from more experienced clinicians.

However, the value of the task and the reward for the patient make this endeavor worth the effort. The essence of neurocritical care is the provision of patient- and brain-specific care to improve clinical outcomes. Our current knowledge of secondary injury and deterioration suggests that patient management directed by physical examination and periodic radiographic imaging has severe limitations. A neurocritical care unit that is not seeking to provide brain-specific care can expect outcomes similar to those of a well-run general critical care unit (10). Notwithstanding the extra work required, members of the clinical team tend to derive significant job satisfaction and intellectual fulfillment from participation in the provision of MMM-directed care.

INNOVATION AND COMPATIBILITY IN A SMALL MARKET

Ischemic stroke, traumatic brain injury, and brain hemorrhage account for a sizable portion of our nation's morbidity and mortality. Despite this reality, few of these patients are cared for by neurointensivists. This is due to the relative youth of the subspecialty, as well as the paucity of physicians dedicated to this field. There are approximately 500 United Council of Neurologic Subspecialties board-certified neurointensivists throughout the world (11). In the United States, accredited neurocritical care training programs are graduating fellows at a rate of only 35 to 50 physicians per year. Neurointensivists have traditionally been the primary users and advocates for MMM, so the demand for neuromonitoring devices has lagged behind their potential utility. For many of the neuromonitoring devices, the market is supplied by only a single commercial vendor. The resulting lack of free-market competition has had impact on device costs, service, and scientific innovation. Many of the available neuromonitoring products also have limited compatibility with bedside monitors and other neuromonitoring systems. The lack of a common platform increases technology expenses and nursing burden.

Recent demand for neuromonitoring has increased and industry interest has followed. Given the size of the patient population served, the potential for continued growth is promising. The recent national trends toward disease-specific hospital accreditation and disease-directed hospital triage are likely to make cutting edge technology and neurocritical care programs top priorities for hospital strategic planning (12,13). This movement is also likely to support the escalation of neuromonitoring.

THE FUTURE OF MULTIMODAL MONITORING: BEYOND THE BASICS

Many neuromonitoring techniques are currently being utilized at their most basic levels. The obstacles associated with assessment of raw cEEG data are being addressed with improved event detection software and greater utilization of compressed spectral array analysis. Similarly, the standard microdialysis analyte profiles of glucose, lactate, pyruvate, glutamate, and glycerol can be expanded to include quantification of anticonvulsants, chemotherapeutic agents, inflammatory markers, and cytokines (14,15). Expansion of neuromonitoring capacity is a key to growth and widened utilization.

Multimodal Monitoring as a Piece of the Clinical Puzzle

MMM is not the answer. Rather, it is part of the answer. In the quest to improve patient outcomes, a practitioner would not abandon the neurologic examination because it fails to provide all of the information necessary to care for the patient. Instead, the knowledge gained from the examination is compared to laboratory data, imaging, vital signs, and other contributing information. At times, some of the data appear contradictory or lead to false conclusions. This may be a result of poor specificity or misinterpretation of the data. We have been using our hands, blood draws, and sphygmomanometer to practice MMM for decades. We have grown accustomed to accepting the limitations of these "monitoring strategies." Our expectations for neuromonitoring should be similarly reasonable. Secondary injury is mediated by dozens of biochemical pathways that are influenced by dozens of modulatory biomarkers (16). It should not surprise us when fastidious monitoring of one mechanism of injury fails to prevent clinical worsening. Nor should this result devalue the importance of what was discovered.

The complexity of the postinjured brain requires comprehensive and complementary strategies for successful monitoring. MMM approaches to patient care are inevitably more descriptive than unimodal monitoring. Regional monitors may fail to provide information relevant to a remote portion of the brain (17). Global monitors often lack the capacity to detect a local event lost in the noise of the aggregate signal (18). A cerebral blood flow monitor may verify adequate perfusion but tell nothing of the accumulation of oxygen-free radicals. A cEEG may exclude epileptic events, but provide little information regarding the brain's auto regulatory state. As a result, the value of these monitors is optimized when used in concert. While current monitoring protocols recognize and account for this observation, there is still much to be learned regarding the appropriate regional placement of monitors and the most effective combinations of neuromonitoring devices for each disease state.

These unanswered questions should not dissuade the team from MMM implementation. In our limited understanding of monitoring and secondary injury, we have already seen that clinical deterioration can be reversed and that monitoring provides us with insights that influence our approach to therapeutic intervention (19).

WHAT DO YOU SEE?

If we take the effort to monitor a patient via MMM, we should view our data in a format that allows causal relationships and data associations to be discovered. The human mind is ill equipped to draw correlations between data points and consequence from a tabular format. Graphically presented data that is time matched and sequenced allow for clearer comparisons (see Figure 12.1). The incompatibility of several neuromonitoring systems can limit implementation of this type of data display. Recently, several vendors have marketed data integration systems with these display goals in mind. Such a system is essential to sort through the myriad of possible interactions among patient variables.

Data must be organized so that combinations of data points known to influence each other (temperature, ICP, ischemic markers) are able to be viewed simultaneously. Likewise, data from multiple monitors must be presented in a manner that allows recognition of physiologically pertinent variability of each. For example, changes in interstitial glucose concentrations will not be recognized if these data share a graphical scale and plot with LPR. The scale of each data element should illuminate deviations from the norm.

CHALLENGES

All considered, there are numerous challenges to initiating and maintaining an efficient and productive MMM program. The neurocritical care community has taken strides to address these issues and define the purpose of each device as a clinical tool. Outcome-related

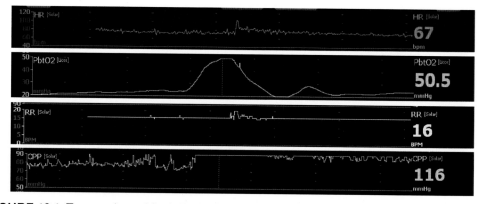

FIGURE 12.1 Temporal graphical display of data with each parameter represented in physiologically appropriate scale.

research with MMM-directed protocols are currently underway. The physiologic rationale for MMM makes the prospects of favorable conclusions promising for these studies. The topics addressed in this chapter are pivotal in determining the direction of MMM globally. Their relevance is equally pertinent to the success of each individual MMM program.

REFERENCES

1. Skjoth-Rasmussen J, Schulz M, Kristensen SR et al. Delayed neurological deficits detected by an ischemic pattern in the extracellular cerebral metabolites in patients with aneurismal subarachnoid hemorrhage. *J Neurosurg.* 2004;100:8–15.
2. Vespa PM. O'Phelan K. McArthur D. et al. Pericontusional brain tissue exhibits persistent elevation of lactate/pyruvate ratio independent of cerebral perfusion pressure. *Critical Care Medicine.* 2007;35(4):1153–1160.
3. Valadka AB, Gopinath SP, Contant CF, et al. Relationship of brain tissue PO_2 to outcome after severe head injury. *Critical Care Medicine.* 1998;26(9):1576–1581.
4. Clermont G, Kong L, Weissfeld LA, et al. The effect of pulmonary artery catheter use on costs and long-term outcomes of acute lung injury. *PLoS One* 2011;6(7):e22512.
5. Chesnut RM, Temkin N, Carney N, et al. A trial of intracranial-pressure monitoring in traumatic brain injury. *N Engl J Med.* 2012;367(26):2471–2481.
6. Schmidt JM, Wartenberg KE, Fernandez A, et al. Frequency and clinical impact of asymptomatic cerebra infarction due to vasospasm after subarachnoid hemorrhage. *J Neurosurg.* 2008;109:1052–1059.
7. Guidelines for the management of severe traumatic brain injury. *J Neurotrauma.* 2007;24 (Suppl 1):S1–S106.
8. Morgenstern LB, Hemphill JC, Anderson C, et al. Guidelines for the Management of Spontaneous *Intracerebral Hemorrhage.* Stroke 2010;41:2108–2129.
9. Connolly ES, Rabinstein AA, Carhuapoma JR, et al. Guidelines for the Management of Aneursymal Subarachnoid Hemmorhage. a guideline for Healthcare Professionals From the American Heart Association/American Stroke Association. *Stroke.* 2012;43(6):1711–1737.
10. Josephson SA, Douglas V, Lawton MT, et al. Improvement in intensive care unit outcomes in patients with subarachnoid hemorrhage after initiation of neurointensivist co-management. *J Neurosurg.* 2010;112:626–630.
11. UCNS Congratulates Diplomates in Neurocritical Care. Available: http://www.ucns.org/globals/axon/assets/10301.pdf. Date accessed December 31, 2013.
12. Rosner J, Nuno M, Miller C, et al. Subarachnoid Hemorrhage Patients: To Transfer or Not to Transfer? *Neurosurgery.* 2013;60 (Suppl 1):98–101.
13. Dion JE. Management of ischemic stroke in the next decade: stroke centers of excellence. *J Vasc Interv Radiol.* 2004;15:S133–S141.
14. Kanafy KA, Grobelny B, Fernandez L, et al. Brain interstitial fluid TNF-ɑ after subarachnoid hemorrhage. *J Neurol Sci.* 2010;291:69–73.
15. Tisdall M, Russo S, Sen J, et al. Free phenytoin concentration measurement in brain extracellular fluid: a pilot study. *Br J Neurosurg.* 2006;20(5):285–289.
16. Mcilvoy LH. The effect of hypothermia and hyperthermia on acute brain injury. *AACN Clin Issues.* 2005;16(4):488–500.
17. Miller, CM, Palestrant D. Distribution of delayed ischemic neurological deficits after aneurysmal subarachnoid hemorrhage and implications for regional monitoring. *Clin Neu and Neurosurg.* 2012;114:545–549.
18. Gopinath SP, Valadka AB, Uzura M, et al. Comparison of jugular venous oxygen saturation and brain tissue PO_2 as monitors of cerebral ischemia after head injury. *Crit Care Med.* 1999;27(11):2337–2345.
19. Sarrafzadeh AS, Haux D, Ludemann L, et al. Cerebral ischemia in aneurysmal subarachnoid hemorrhage: a correlative microdialysis-PET study. *Stroke.* 2004;35(3):638–643.

Index